OBESITY...

It's *NOT* what *YOU THINK* it is!

RICHARD FAST

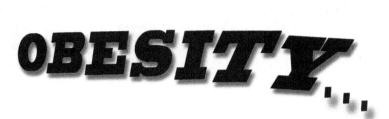

OBESITY...

It's **NOT** what **YOU THINK** it is!

ISBN: 978-0-9879193-9-7

29 DAYS Publishing Inc.

TABLE OF CONTENTS

INTRODUCTION 6

PART 1 – THE PROBLEM

Key Facts from the World Health Organization 9
Global Obesity! How Did It Happen? 10
What Caused Indiscriminate Weight Gain? 11
What Common Factor Could Cause Nationwide Weight Gain? 13
Americans Are Much Sicker Than They Realize 14

PART 11 – THE CULPRIT

The Birth of the Modern Diet 18
The Critical Ingredients of America's New Diet: Cheap, Fast and Convenient 19
Give Us Quick, Easy and Convenient: America Makes a Faustian Deal 20
Big Food Delivered ... and Then Some 21
We Can't Win a War If We Don't Know Our Enemy 22
The Scorpion and The Frog: A Tale of Modern Capitalism 23
To Understand Big Business ... Follow the Money 23
The Frank Statement: Big Tobacco Takes No Prisoners 24
A Modern Tale of David and Goliath 25
The Big Business Playbook: Sow Doubt, Deceive and Delay 26
Big Business and the Interchangeable Script of Denial 27
The Personal Responsibility Script 27
Tobacco Industry Promises Self-Regulation 28
Tobacco Exploits New Markets 28
Big Food Pursues Self-Regulatory Authority 30
Trends and Results ... The Tale of the Tape 32
The Magician's Sleight of Hand: Corporate Social Responsibility 35
The Playbook: Influence Government and Key Organizations 36
Smart Choices Program: How to Eat Your Cake AND Be Healthy Too! 36
We Don't Recommend ALL Junk Food, Just the Healthiest Junk Food 39
Coca-Cola Employs the Best "Scientific" Studies Money Can Buy! 40

Scientific Studies that Disprove Scientific Studies! 41
Coca-Cola Gets Caught with Its Hand in the "Selective-Science" Cookie Jar 42
Coke Promises to Come Clean 43
How to Get a Planet Fat: Create Food Addictions … One Door at a Time 45
Brazil Gets Hooked 45
Over Fed and Under Nourished 48
Profits are Booming … All is Well 49
Malaysia Drinks Industry Kool-Aid, Becoming the Fattest Nation in Asia 50
Smart Choices Labeling … Déjà vu All Over Again? 51
Dr. Tee's "Work" Speaks for Itself 52
The Takeaway 53

PART III – THE CAUSE

Is Global Obesity the Result of a Single Cause? 57
The Birth of Ultra-Processed Food and the Simultaneous Rise in Obesity 58
Brazil's Obesity Detective Identifies the Killer 59
Brazil Introduces a "Practical" and Revolutionary Food Guide 60
"Processed" Food is a Critical Component to Our Health 61
The NOVA Classification of Processed Food 62
The Unsavoury Truth of Ultra-Processed "Food" 63
UPFs: Tasty, Cheap, Ubiquitous and Oh So Profitable 65
Why Are Ultra-Processed Foods SO Hard to Resist? 66
Understanding "Real" Food 66
Understanding Ultra-Processed Food 67
Ultra-Processed Food is More Than a Language; It's a Complete Science! 67
Are Ultra-Processed Foods Addictive? 68
Ultra-Processed Food – Habit or Addiction? 68
3 "Scientific" Studies Confirm Ultra-Processed Food Drives Obesity 70
What Would It Take to Change Your Mind? 70
Study #1 A True Scientist Changes His Mind 71
Researcher Finds the Evidence … Surprising 72
Study #2 How to Lose 12-Pounds of FAT, Without Counting a Single Calorie! ... 78
Stop Counting Calories and Lose Weight? 81
Study #3 What Are We Feeding Our Kids? 83
Eating Junk Food for One Month Took Ten Years Off My Life! 83
It's Not a Lack of Moral Fibre, It's About What's Available to Eat 83

A Candid Interview with the Food and Drink Federation 88

The Takeaway 89

PART IV – THE CURE

The Cure for Obesity is Not to Focus on Weight; It's to Focus on Health 93

There's No Such Thing as a Healthy Weight, Only a Healthy Person 94

We've Been Led to Believe (Wrongly) that Being "Overweight" is a Direct Cause of Premature Death 95

Could You Be Obese and Not Even Know It? 98

All We Need is a Good Pair of Walking Shoes 102

To Reverse Global Obesity, We Must Change Our Perspective 105

"You" Have to Change, BEFORE "You" Can Change 106

I'll Change … But NOT Today! 107

Overcoming the Circular Dilemma 108

At Last, I Could Clearly See What I was Giving Up … Nothing! 110

What About Regression? Why Was This Time Different? 110

Why is it So Difficult to Change Our Deep-seated Habits and Beliefs? 111

Want Lasting Change? Forget About Willpower and Teeth-Gritted Effort 111

Changing Our Perspective of Food 112

How Should We View Big Food and the Ultra-Processed Food It's Peddling?.... 112

What Happens to Your Body When You Eat Ultra-Processed Food? 113

You Can Lose Weight, Eat All Your Favorite Foods, AND Enjoy a Lifetime of Health Without Counting a Single Calorie 114

What Do You Find Acceptable? 116

Some Closing Thoughts 118

ABOUT ME 123

OTHER BOOKS 125

Introduction

Our relationship with food is broken. Consequently, so is our health.

Until recently, food was not only treasured for sustenance and survival; it meant comfort and sharing, a celebration of life.

But that's all changed. Food is no longer food. For many people, food has become both friend and foe. While we cherish it for sustenance, we resent it for making us fat. We find solace in chowing down "comfort food" after a long day and then silently berate ourselves for lacking willpower.

We don't go to a supermarket and buy food; we buy brightly coloured, cleverly designed packages, each heralding its healthful benefits.

When we talk about food, we speak in terms of carbs, fats, proteins, calories, and antioxidants.

We're inundated with endless admonitions to eat less fat, more fat, go organic, Paleo, ketogenic, plant-based, and God only knows what else.

The media has become a never-ending stream of studies, warnings, contradictions, conspiracies, and retractions. What was good for us a few years ago suddenly isn't. What wasn't unexpectedly is.

How is it that we humans, who are exponentially "smarter" than all other species, can be so confounded by something as natural and straightforward as food? No animal in the wild has a problem with obesity, or diabetes or the host of other non-communicable diseases that face humans.

OBESITY... *It's NOT what YOU THINK it is!*

So, what's going on? How have "we," the most intelligent species on this planet, lost our way?

This book is not about dieting and weight loss (although it will show you how to lose weight in a surprisingly simple way), it's a book about health; how we lose it and how we can get it back.

The obesity pandemic is no illusion. We urgently need to wake up from our "food" induced trance because whether we realize it or not, we're in a fight for the highest stakes possible ... our health and the future health of our children.

"What an extraordinary achievement for a civilization; to have developed the one diet that reliably makes its people sick!"

~Michael Pollan

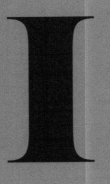

part I

The Problem

*__Problem__ ~ A situation that's difficult
to deal with or control.*

Merriam-Webster

For the entirety of life on this planet, obesity was unimaginable. In fact, most creatures are hungry most of the time. Our problem is different.

We are the first species to create the absurd paradox of being overweight and undernourished at the same time, resulting in a rising obesity pandemic that spans the globe.

Key Facts from World Health Organization

➡ In 1986, 1 in 200 adults in America were morbidly obese; by 2004, the figure was 1 in 50. By 2017 it was 1 in 5. (1)

➡ Worldwide obesity has nearly tripled between 1975 and 2016.

➡ In 1976–1980, only 6.2% of young adults had so-called obesity (BMI [Body Mass Index] of 30 or higher). In 2017-2018 nearly 33% of this age group had a BMI in excess of 30. (2)

➡ Among children and adolescents aged 5-19 obesity has risen from just 4% in 1975 to over 18% in 2016. (3) In 2019, 19 % of youths aged 2 to 19 were obese, and just a year later, it rose to 22%. (13)

➡ Most of the world's population live in countries where overweight kills more people than underweight. (3)

Global Obesity! How Did It Happen?

For thousands of years, human body weight stayed remarkably stable. Throughout adulthood, we consumed no more than the food we needed to burn. People who were overweight stood out from the general population. Millions of calories passed through our bodies, yet with rare exceptions, our weight neither rose nor fell by any significant amount. A perfect biological system seemed to be at work. Then, something changed. (4)

It seems we can almost pinpoint the beginning of global obesity in the U.S.A. to 1975.

1975 Obesity Begins in USA

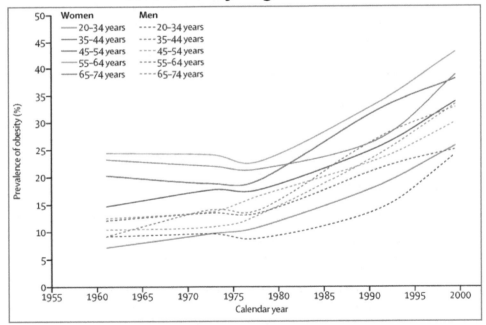

Figure: Prevalence of obesity, by age and sex.
Data from US Centers for Disease Control and Prevention,
National Health and Examination Surveys (1960–2000) (5)

OBESITY It's NOT what YOU THINK it is!

Once obesity began, it increased year after year with astonishing increments; what's more, it spread among the entire population showing little preference for age, gender or ethnicity.

What Caused Indiscriminate Weight Gain?

Theories abound.

Some suggest a decline in manual labour. However, according to a paper in the *International Journal of Surgery,* adults working in unskilled manual professions are four times more likely to be classified as morbidly obese compared to those in professional employment. (1)

Others say it results from a sedentary lifestyle, which seems to make sense; we drive rather than walk, ride elevators and escalators in place of climbing stairs. Video games replaced outdoor play.

However, in a study published in 2012, anthropologist Herman Pontzer went to Tanzania to study the Hadza, one of the few remaining hunter-gatherer tribes. He fully expected to find evidence supporting the prevailing theories that obesity results from inactivity.

For 11 days, Pontzer and his team tracked the movements and energy expenditure of 13 men and 17 women ages 18 to 75, using a technique called doubly labelled water – the best-known way to measure the carbon dioxide we expel throughout the day.

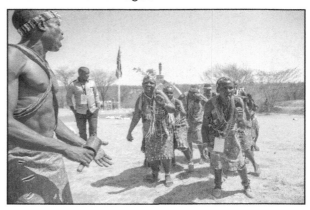

The results were astonishing.

While the hunter-gatherers were physically active and lean, they burned the same

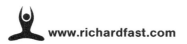

number of calories as the average American or European, even after the researchers controlled for body size.

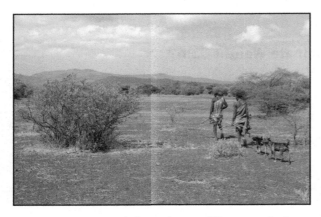

How could the hunting, foraging Hadza burn the same amount of energy as sedentary Westerners?

According to Pontzer, "They don't overeat, so they don't become obese." (6)

A paper in the *International Journal of Epidemiology* finds that corrected for body size; there is no difference between the number of calories burned by people in rich countries and those in poor ones, where subsistence agriculture remains the norm. (7)

An overwhelming number of studies suggest that exercise, while crucial to other aspects of good health, plays a minor role in regulating our weight. Many researchers propose it plays no role at all as the more we exercise, the hungrier we get. (8)

In another theory, an international survey of more than 300 policymakers in 2014 reported that more than 90% believed personal motivation was a powerful influence in the rise of obesity. (9)

How a large majority of a diverse population can collectively lose their willpower isn't explained.

And yet another theory suggests obesity is the result of genetics. However, if intrauterine (in uterus) exposures played a significant role, one would have to hypothesize a time lag of about 70 years for babies born in 1910, 60 years for those born in 1920, and so on. It's implausible. Changes in genetic predisposition do not occur over a few years, nor

OBESITY... *It's NOT what YOU THINK it is!*

do they affect all age groups simultaneously. (10)

Under closer examination of all the prevailing theories, from sedentary lifestyles to genetics to a lack of personal motivation, none can explain indiscriminate population-wide weight gain.

What is the One Common Factor That Could Cause Nationwide Weight Gain?

Food. More specifically, it's the "food-like" substances we're eating. It begins to make perfect sense when we look at the consumption figures in more detail.

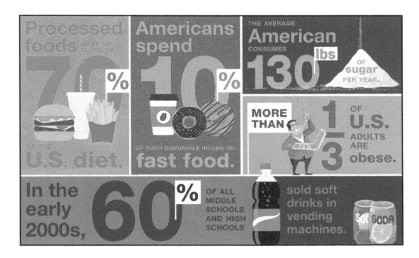

One of the most comprehensive research studies on the obesity pandemic showed that it had swept the globe, including regions that have historically had food shortages, like Africa.

The study, compiled by the *Institute for Health Metrics and Evaluation* at the University of Washington, looked at 195 countries, essentially the world's population, finding that rates of obesity at least doubled in 73 countries from 1980 to 2015, and "continuously increased in most other

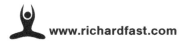

countries." The study defined obese as a body mass index of 30 or higher and overweight as a B.M.I. from 25 to 29. (11)

By those measures, nearly 604 million adults and 108 million children worldwide are obese.

And worse, obesity rates among children are rising faster in many countries than among adults.

The study did not go deeply into the causes of obesity. Still, the authors said the growing accessibility of inexpensive, nutrient-poor packaged foods was probably a significant factor, and the general slowdown in physical activity was probably not.

According to Dr. Ashkan Afshin, the lead author of the study:

"We have more processed food, more energy-dense food, more intense marketing of food products, and these products are more available and more accessible," he added. "The food environment seems to be the main driver of obesity."

American's Are Much Sicker Than They Realize

More than 100 million adults — almost half the entire adult population — have pre-diabetes or diabetes. Cardiovascular disease afflicts about 122 million people and causes roughly 840,000 deaths each year, or about 2,300 deaths each day. Three in four adults are overweight or obese. (12)

More Americans are sick than are healthy. We need to answer the question;

What is making us so sick?

The rest of this book will explore how we got ourselves into this obesity predicament and, more importantly, how we can get out!

References

1. Agha, M., Agha, R., "The Rising Prevalence of Obesity: Part A: Impact on Public Health," International Journal of Surgery, August;2017: 2 (7)
2. Ellison-Barnes, A., Johnson, S., Gudzune, K., "Trends in Obesity Prevalence Among Adults Aged 18 Through 25 Years, 1976-2018," JAMA 2021;326(20):2073-2074
3. Obesity and Overweight, World Health Organization, June 9, 2021
4. Kessler, D., "The End of Overeating: Taking Control of the Insatiable American Appetite," Rodale Inc. New York, NY, 2009
5. Data from US Centers for Disease Control and Prevention, National Health and Examination Surveys (1960-2000)
6. Pontzer, H., et. al., "Hunter-Gatherer Energetics and Human Obesity," PLOS ONE, July 25, 2012
7. Luke, A., Cooper, R. S., "Physical Activity Does Not Influence Obesity Risk: Time to Clarify the Public Health Message," International Journal of Epidemiology, Vol 42, Issue 6, December 2013)1831-1836
8. Thomas, D.M. et al., "Why Do Individuals Not Lose More Weight from an Exercise Intervention at a Defined Dose? An Energy Balance Analysis," National Institute of Health, Obes Rev. 2012 Oct;13(10): 835-847
9. European Association for the Study of Obesity. Obesity Perception and Policy, Multi-Country Review and Survey of Policymakers. May 2014
10. Rodgers, A., Woodward, A., Boyd Swinburn, W. H., "Prevalence Trends Tell Us What Did Not Precipitate the US Obesity Epidemic," The Lancet, Vol. 3, April 2018
11. The GBD 2015 Obesity Collaborators, "Effects of Overweight and Obesity in 195 Countries over 25 Years," The New England Journal of Medicine, 2017; 377:13-27
12. Mozaffarian, D., Glickman, D., "Our Food is Killing Too Many of Us; Improving American nutrition would make the biggest impact on our health care," New York Times, August 26, 2019
13. Neuman, S., "Children and Teens Gained Weight at An Alarming Rate During the Pandemic, the CDC Says," NPR, September, 17, 2021

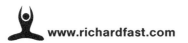

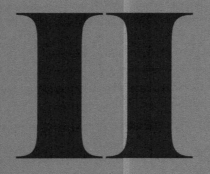

part II

The Culprit

__Culprit__ ~ One guilty of a crime or a fault; the source or cause of a problem.
Merriam-Webster

The global obesity pandemic is a direct result of *what* we eat – too much ultra-processed, nutrient-void garbage.

That may not be surprising, but it raises a question; If we *"know"* the food we eat is destroying our health, why don't we do anything about it? Why do we continue consuming our present diet? What's causing us to follow along in lockstep as if we were drug-induced automatons? What's enabling our complicity to "willfully" grow fatter and less healthy year after year?

To answer these questions, we need to go back in time, but not too far, just enough to see ...

The Birth of the "Modern" Diet

Before the industrial age, most of the food we ate was locally raised or grown. In the late nineteenth century, with the advent of railroads, food began to be mass-produced. Since it could be transported over a long distance, it significantly reduced dependence on food from the local farm.

With the dawn of the 20th century, America began to wake up to a revolutionary new breakfast – processed cereal. It was a radical departure from the traditional staples like bacon, eggs, and porridge. Cereals were not only lighter and easier to digest, but they were also wonderfully convenient. Pour it out of a box, add some cold milk and breakfast is served. A perfect solution for the men and women who were adapting to the quicker pace of a growing industrialized nation.

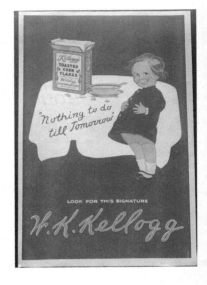

As Americans began to consume processed foods in mass quantity, competition grew fierce. Food began to be identified as a brand. With the irresistible combination of health claims and convenience, Kellogg's, Post, and other food manufacturers began to change how America thought about food.

The 1920s saw the introduction of techniques for freezing food and the invention of preservatives, which revolutionized storage and preparation. Processed and packaged foods were quickly becoming a cornerstone of the American diet.

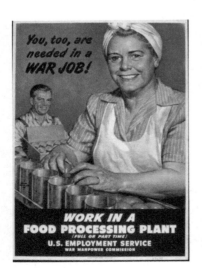

World War II created a much greater need for processed foods. The food industry began producing convenience foods such as dehydrated juice, Spam, instant coffee, and cake mix to feed America's soldiers.

Following World War II, the food companies turned their attention to the American housewife. Processed foods were suddenly transformed to become "packaged cuisine."

The 1950s brought television, superhighways and heat-and-serve prepared foods. As millions of women entered the workforce, Mom was no longer at home to cook. But now, thanks to

OBESITY... *It's NOT what YOU THINK it is!*

TV dinners, when Mom was asked the age-old question, "What's for dinner?", she could say, "What would you like?"

What more could American Moms want? TV dinners were cheap, convenient and they came in endless varieties. Pop them in the oven, and 25 minutes later, you could enjoy a full meal while feasting on the new national pastime; television. (1)

The Critical Ingredients of America's New Diet: Cheap, Fast and Convenient

With the advent of superhighways, commuting, suburbs and two-car garages, America was on the go. Fast food was both inevitable and wildly successful. It represented a seismic shift in America's lifestyle. Regardless of age, race, or economic background, Americans began to gorge on pizza, tacos, burgers, and bagels.

We weren't just hooked on the taste; we expected endless variety and increasing convenience.

By the 1980s, we drove to gigantic supermarkets to load up on a week's supply of ready-to-eat foods. New products sprung forth with metronomic regularity.

Canned, bottled, frozen or dried, highly processed foods became the bulk of our new diet. With each package promising to meet all our "essential" needs, we were seduced to dump fresh food and home-prepared meals for a "better" life of ease, comfort, and "nutrition."

The food was awful, delicious and addictive!

The hook was set!

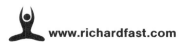

Give Us Quick, Easy, and Convenient:
America Makes a Faustian Deal

The story of Faust and his deal-with-the-Devil has an uncanny similarity to our "negotiated" arrangement with Big Food Companies.

As the story goes, Doctor Faust, was a scholar, who was bored, depressed, and frustrated with man's limited knowledge. So after a failed attempt to take his own life, he called on the Devil in search of a life of wisdom and hedonism. Faust tells the Devil that the only God he serves is his own appetite.

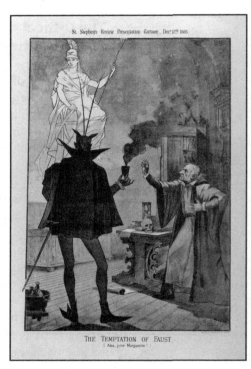

THE TEMPTATION OF FAUST
(Alas, poor Marguerite!)

Hearing that, the Devil sends his representative, Mephistopheles, to negotiate a deal.

Mephistopheles offers him the opportunity to sample every possible delight;

"Grasp at what you want. Your palate shall be sated, your nostrils sweetly stimulated, your sense of touch exhilarated."

"For twenty-four years, you shall have your heart's desire, but in the end, the Devil will have the right to claim your soul. Is it a deal?"

Faust agrees and immediately makes use of Mephistopheles in various ways. Through him, Faust acquires a harem of beautiful women, enjoys adventurous travels and learns the art of magic.

OBESITY *It's NOT what YOU THINK it is!*

But the Devil would have his due. On the last evening of the agreed term, amid a terrible storm, the Devil tears the doctor's body apart, claims his soul and carries him off to hell.

Today, a "Faustian Bargain" is considered any deal made for short-term gain with *unexpected* long-term costs. From credit cards to fast food, we tend to make Faustian deals with regularity. We'll opt for immediate pleasure ignoring the consequences of tomorrow until tomorrow. But tomorrow always arrives, and it has a nasty habit of coming much sooner than we thought.

Without realizing it, we made a Faustian deal with the Big Food companies. Our food is rich and succulent, salty and crispy, sweet and smooth. It comes in endless variety, it's available everywhere, and it's so tasty we can't stop eating it.

Big Food Delivered ... and Then Some!

For many years everyone was happy with our "deal". We got blissfully addicted to gorging on cheap, delicious food while the manufacturers got blissfully addicted to "ginormous" profits.

And then the cracks began to appear. A US government survey on data collected from 1988 to 1991 revealed that one-third of the population aged twenty to seventy-four weighed too much. In fewer than a dozen years, an additional 20 million Americans had joined the ranks of the overweight.

The results were consistent across the board — among men and women, young and old, black and white. The rate of obesity in America had exploded! [2]

Here's the thing, whenever a deal seems too good to be true ... it is. We thoughtlessly gave the food industry carte blanche for our diet in exchange for convenience, variety, and flavour. We got everything we bargained for and more.

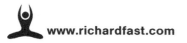

We got "food-like" substances that are cheap, delicious, and addictive, all for the low, low, price of our health, independence, and "enjoyment" of food.

Food, after all, is more than a means of subsistence. It's more than scarfing something down in the car, at meetings or while walking down a sidewalk. Food has traditionally been an integral part of our culture. It's what embodies the "human experience." It's been about sharing, cooking, and celebrating together. We've lost so much.

We can't seem to wake up from our food-induced coma and say "no more" to this deal. If we did it may mean a little less convenience and a little more cost in terms of time, but that's a small price to pay to restore all that we've lost.

At present, our collective well-being is in serious trouble. Make no mistake, we're at war. We're in a fight for the highest stakes possible, our health and the future health of our children.

We Can't Win a War If We Don't Know Our Enemy

Large, publicly held companies have one purpose: Profit. In fact, it's a legal and moral obligation to their shareholders.

Nobel laureate Milton Friedman wrote in his classic work, *Capitalism and Freedom*, "There is one and only one social responsibility of business – to use its resources and engage in activities designed to increase its profit so long as it stays within the rules of the game, which is to say, engages in open and free competition, without deception or fraud." (3)

In *Appetite for Profit*, Michele Simon writes, " ... under our current economic system it's not a corporation's job to protect public health ... in fact, managers who willfully allow the bottom line to suffer to protect the public good can be sued by company shareholders for breach of their legal obligations. (4)

OBESITY... *It's NOT what YOU THINK it is!*

The Scorpion and The Frog:
A Tale of Modern Capitalism

Surviving in Wall Street's world requires a *particular nature*; you either got *it*, or you don't. Wall Street expects more than just profits; they want an increase in shareholder value every quarter. To convince customers to buy your product in a ruthlessly competitive market, you'd better have "it"!

"It" brings to mind the classic fable of the scorpion who desperately needed to cross a river. Unable to swim, the scorpion cunningly approaches a frog and pleads, "Mr. Frog, can you carry me across the river on your back?"

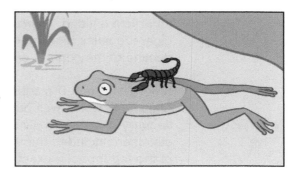

"I hardly think so, "replies the frog, "you'll sting me."

"Why would I do that?" asked the scorpion. "If I sting you, we'd both drown."

The logic proved sound so the frog agreed.

The scorpion climbed onto the frog's back, and together they set off. Just as they neared the middle of the river, the scorpion twitched his tail and stung the frog. Mortally wounded, the frog cried out: "Why did you sting me? Don't you realize we're both going to die?"

"I couldn't help it," said the scorpion, "*it's* just my nature."

To Understand Big Business ... Follow the Money

We're all familiar with the history of the tobacco industry and its ruthless disregard for social responsibility. But as we'll see, the "nature" of the tobacco industry and the "nature" of the food industry are indistinguishable:

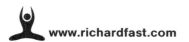

Both industries are dominated by a few major players that manufacture and market products to create habits, addictions, and life-long customers. (5)

The Frank Statement: Big Tobacco Takes No Prisoners

In December 1953, the CEOs of the major tobacco companies met secretly in New York City. Their purpose was to counter the damage from studies linking smoking to lung cancer. A year earlier, *Reader's Digest* — then the public's leading source of medical information — had printed an article entitled *"Cancer by the Carton."* After it appeared, cigarette sales plummeted for two years, the first such decline of the century except during the Great Depression.

From that "secret" meeting came the now-classic *Frank Statement*, which was published in 448 newspapers on January 4, 1954. To give the industry a human face, the statement included the signatures of the top tobacco executives and assured Americans that *"we accept an interest in people's health as a basic responsibility, paramount to every other consideration in our business."* Furthermore, they promised that *"we always have and always will cooperate closely with those whose task it is to safeguard the public's health."* (6)

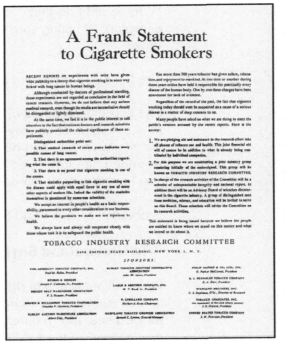

Everything was at stake. The tobacco industry would do anything to prevent, or at least delay, shifts in public opinion that would permit a barrage of legislative, regulatory, and legal actions that would erode sales and profits.

A Modern Tale of David and Goliath

Tobacco companies would protect their turf at all costs. They employed some of the most prestigious law firms in the country and commanded the allegiance of a significant section of Congress. It also had access to the services of widely admired public figures, ranging from Prime Minister Margaret Thatcher to Senator Howard Baker. With its limitless resources and a corporate culture that was aggressively defensive, the industry perceived threats everywhere and responded to them ferociously. They were untouchable. (7)

To David Kessler, it didn't matter. As Commissioner of the U.S. Food and Drug Administration (FDA) from 1990 to 1997, he systematically and methodically exposed the tobacco *Playbook*. He focused on collecting evidence of what the companies knew. He revealed the master plan and script that directed industry executives, lobbyists, lawyers, scientists, and government officials friendly to the industry. (8)

In his book, *A Question of Intent*, Kessler wrote:

> Devised in the 1950s and '60s, the tobacco industry's strategy was embodied in a script written by the lawyers. Every tobacco company executive in the public eye was told to learn the script backwards and forwards, no deviation allowed. The basic premise was simple — smoking had not been proved to cause cancer. Not proven, not proven, not proven — this would be stated insistently and repeatedly. Inject a thin wedge of doubt, create controversy, never deviate from the prepared lines. It was a simple plan, and it worked. "It made us look like horses' asses," said Veritas (*industry informer*). But the industry never lost a case, and that was all that mattered to them. (7)

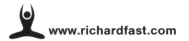

The Big Business Playbook: Sow Doubt, Deceive and Delay

Big Tobacco refined the tactics of control, but the script has been played out by powerful elites for hundreds if not thousands of years for one reason ... it works.

Big Food not only copied the *Playbook*, it tweaked the recipe and came up with its own formula:

Big Food Companies Playbook

➤ Focus on personal responsibility as the cause of the nation's unhealthy diet.

➤ Raise fears that government action usurps personal freedom.

➤ Vilify critics with totalitarian language, characterizing them as the food police, leaders of a nanny state, and even "food fascists," and accuse them of desiring to strip people of their civil liberties.

➤ Criticize studies that hurt the industry as "junk science."

➤ Emphasize physical activity over diet.

➤ State there are no good or bad foods; hence no food or food type (soft drinks, fast foods, etc.) should be targeted.

➤ Plant doubt when concerns are raised about the industry by funding research to produce desired results.

➤ Use the courts to challenge critics and unfavourable regulations.

➤ Appear to be a socially responsible corporate citizen. [8, 9]

OBESITY *It's NOT what YOU THINK it is!*

Big Business and the Interchangeable Script of Denial

The Playbook has been a critical strategy for many industries; hire consultants to skew scientific literature and sow doubt to keep the public confused. It's worked for global warming, second-hand smoke, asbestos, lead, plastics, and many other toxic materials. Industry executives pay unscrupulous scientists and lobbyists to dispute any evidence contrary to their interests, which they'll label as "junk science." (10)

Likewise, groups and scientists funded by the food industry have disputed whether the prevalence figures for obesity are correct, whether obesity causes disease and whether foods like soft drinks cause harm.

The Personal Responsibility Script

How an issue is framed is a timeless technique of persuasion. Framing a problem as *"personal responsibility"* shifts responsibility from the parties who manufacture and market unsafe products to those who use them.

For example, at the 1996 shareholder's meeting of cigarette and food manufacturer RJR Nabisco, a woman in the audience asked company chairman Charles Harper whether he would want people smoking around his children and grandchildren.

Mr. Harper responded; "If the children don't like to be in a smoky room ... they'll leave."

When the woman stated, "An infant cannot leave a room."

Mr. Harper countered by saying; "At some point, they learn to crawl, okay? And then they begin to walk." (11)

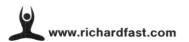

The food companies invoke personal responsibility equally well. In 2004 congressman Ric Keller (R-FL) moved to ban all lawsuits claiming health damages against fast-food restaurants. As he framed it during a CNN interview;

> "We've got to get back to those old-fashioned principles of personal responsibility, of common sense, and get away from this new culture where everybody plays the victim and blames other people for their problems."

When asked about the role of restaurants in contributing to the obesity problem, Steven Anderson, president of the National Restaurant Association stated,

> "Just because we have electricity doesn't mean you have to electrocute yourself."

When asked if eating four times a week at Burger King or McDonald's was healthy?

> "Sure, Anderson says, "if it's balanced, if it's in moderation, if you are getting physical activity." (12)

Food companies argue that they should not be blamed for the obesity pandemic. They're simply responding to consumer demand.

Hmmm, perhaps, but it gets tricky if we're going to chastise a six-year-old for lack of personal responsibility when clever advertisers goaded him or her into collecting all ten toys as advertised! It begs the question; is it a response to consumer demand, or is it the creation of consumer demand?

Tobacco Industry Promises Self-Regulation

The *Frank Statement* of 1954, in which they pledged to cooperate closely with those tasked with safeguarding public health, demonstrates the outright duplicity of the Tobacco industry. In 1991 Tobacco publicly stated their desire for a youth smoking prevention program.

OBESITY... It's NOT what YOU THINK it is!

In 1963 a Brown & Williamson executive wrote, **"We are, then, in the business of selling nicotine, an addictive drug."** (13)

In 1972 a Philip Morris research official wrote, **"The product is nicotine. ... Think of the cigarette pack as a storage container for a day's supply of nicotine."** (14)

In 1974 the CEOs of every major tobacco company in America stood before Congress and, *under oath*, denied believing that smoking caused lung cancer and that nicotine was addictive, despite countless studies (some by their own scientists) showing the opposite. Most troubling was the intentional manipulation of nicotine to increase the addictive potential of cigarettes. (15)

Tobacco Exploits New Markets

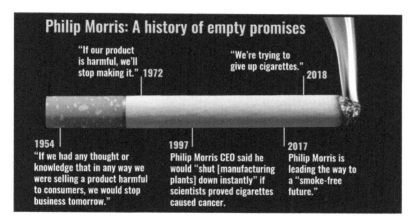

In the early 80's, realizing the jig was up in North America, tobacco companies set off for greener pastures in Latin America. Proclaiming their concern in preventing juvenile smoking, they ran commercials using animated characters (matches) to represent a family having a conversation about adult issues such as smoking. The text read, *"Help your kids make the right choices. Smoking is an adult decision."*

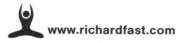

Internal research conducted by Philip Morris Latin America reported that describing smoking as an "adult behaviour" could promote smoking because *if* smoking is an adult behaviour and adolescents want to be adults, adolescents may wish to smoke.

An outside evaluation supported the same conclusion. In fact, it might affect children in ways that would make them more likely to smoke. (16)

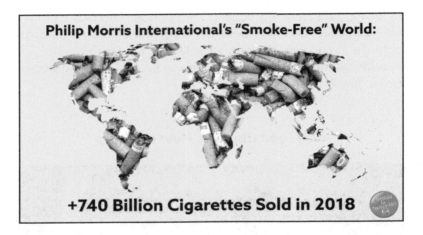

WASHINGTON, DC – Doubling down on its campaign of deception, Philip Morris International – one of the world's largest cigarette manufacturers – recently launched *"The Year of Unsmoke,"* a follow-up to claims that it wants a smoke-free future. It is the height of hypocrisy for Philip Morris to act like it wants to rid the world of cigarettes at the same time that it is aggressively marketing cigarettes across the globe – especially in low- and middle-income countries – and fighting proven policies that reduce smoking and save lives. (17)

Big Food Pursues Self-Regulatory Authority

Not surprising, just like the tobacco industry, the food industry is in full-scale pursuit of self-regulatory authority.

OBESITY,,, It's NOT what YOU THINK it is!

In 2006, the American Beverage Association announced that it would reduce traditional carbonated soft drink sales in schools. However, left untouched was an array of beverages whose sales were increasing (e.g., sports drinks), compared with the conventional carbonated beverages whose sales were declining. (18)

Another example of misleading concern for public health is the announcement by a coalition of major food companies that their child-marketing practices would change.

Food Industry Self-Regulation: Empty Pledges

➤ In 2016, over half of TV ads children viewed from *Children's Food and Beverage Advertising Initiative* (CFBAI), were for brands that companies pledged they would not advertise in child-directed media. Because these ads aired outside of dedicated children's TV programming, companies technically complied with their pledges. But research by the broadcasting regulator Ofcom has shown that children spend 64% of their TV viewing time watching shows not aimed specifically at them.

➤ A study comparing advertising on children's TV channels in 2012 and 2018 found an increase of over 50% in ads for products failing to meet CFBAI nutrition criteria.

➤ Virtually all food and beverage ads during children's programming were for unhealthy products (96% in 2012 and 99% in 2018).

Global Food Research Group, July 2020

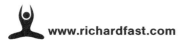

Trends and Results ... The Tale of the Tape

In December 2001, the U.S. Surgeon General issued a *"call to action"* on obesity. The report cited that close to two-thirds of Americans are overweight or obese.

1985: No states had an obesity rate greater than 15%

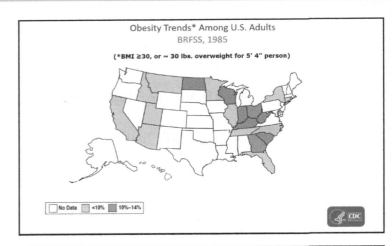

2001: 26 states had obesity rates above 20%

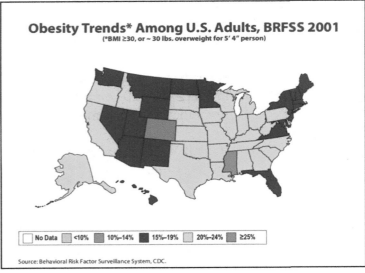

OBESITY... *It's NOT what YOU THINK it is!*

2011: 26 states had obesity rates above 25%

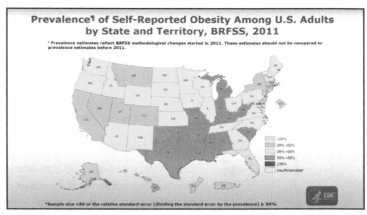

2016: 20 states had obesity rates above 30%, and 5 were above 35%

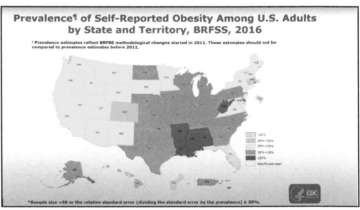

2020: 20 states had obesity rates between 30 and 35% and 15 were above 35%

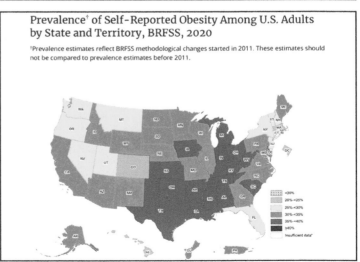

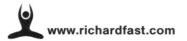

2021 Reports by
World Health Organization and C.D.C.

➤ The worldwide prevalence of obesity nearly tripled between 1975 and 2016.

➤ In 2019, an estimated 38.2 million children under the age of 5 years were overweight or obese in low- and middle-income countries, particularly in urban settings. In Africa, overweight children under 5 have increased by nearly 24% since 2000.

➤ Obesity also appears to be on the increase among U.S. youths. According to the C.D.C., 22 percent of youths ages 2 to 19 were obese in August 2020, up from 19 percent a year earlier, with the most significant increase among children 6 to 11.

Clearly, whatever is being done is either utterly useless, or wildly effective!

OBESITY... *It's NOT what YOU THINK it is!*

The Magician's Sleight of Hand:
Corporate Social Responsibility

For decades, the tobacco industry used perceptions of social responsibility to great effect. They support everything from dance troupes to museums and orchestras. Many charities and group organizations are hard-pressed for funds, so they become vulnerable to the seduction of sponsorship from big businesses (tobacco, food), and they'll show their appreciation in statements of support for their benefactors' good deeds.

Leaders of African American communities faced a genuine conflict: either help the community by accepting money or speak out about the disproportionate toll of tobacco on the health of minority populations. (5, 20)

In 2000, Philip Morris spent $115 million on worthy social causes, including, in addition to the arts, supplying flood victims with clean water and sheltering women who were victims of abuse. The company spent $150 million on a national TV advertising campaign touting its beneficence.

It is noteworthy that such "corporate social responsibility" comes cheap. Philip Morris's spending on good deeds that year constituted one-half of 1 percent of the company's $23 billion in domestic tobacco revenues. (21)

The food industry is equally vested in polishing its image of concern for the public's welfare.

Fast-food restaurants are commonly found in hospitals. Schools remain a branding and sales opportunity for the beverage industry while it pledges to protect children.

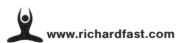

The Playbook: Influence Government and Key Organizations

American Society for Nutrition: The "Best" Nutrition Advice Money Can Buy!

There has been no shortage of examples of industry-funded research producing "scientific" results that defy all credibility, but few could top the duplicity of the American Society for Nutrition (ASN).

The ASN, established in 1928, is the most well-known academic organization in the field of nutrition research; its current membership is about 5,000. ASN is also the publisher of three academic journals, including the *American Journal of Clinical Nutrition*, one of the most respected journals in the field of nutrition. (22)

The ASN Vision: A Healthier World through Evidence-Based Nutrition.

The ASN Mission: To Advance the Science, Education and Practice of Nutrition.

The SMART CHOICES PROGRAM: How to Eat Your Cake AND Be Healthy Too!

In 2009, a new food-labelling campaign called the *Smart Choices Program* (S.C.P.) was conjured up by a coalition of scientists, nutrition educators and ten food companies, including Kraft Foods, ConAgra Foods, Unilever, General Mills, Kellogg's, Tyson Foods and PepsiCo. Companies that participate pay up to $100,000 a year to the Program, with the fee based on total sales of its products that bear the coveted Smart Choices Seal.

More than 2,000 products have received a Smart Choices

OBESITY, *It's NOT what YOU THINK it is!*

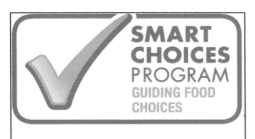

logo, program administrators say. They expect that total to double within months.

The program was designed to set clear public criteria for foods in 19 categories, including cheeses and cheese substitutes; snack foods and sweets; breakfast cereals; fats, oils, and spreads; meals and entrees. The program was to be administered by the A.S.N. in partnership with the non-profit Keystone Center to ensure scientific integrity. The nine-member board of directors included four representatives from the big ten food companies. (24)

According to the Program, any food that met the "scientific" criteria of a "healthy" choice could use the coveted Smart Choices Program label. Sponsors say the logo will help an overweight and overwhelmed public make better food choices in a way that reflects how people really shop.

But it shocked people that *Lucky Charms, Froot Loops, Lunchables Chicken Dunks,* * *Ritz Bits Peanut Butter Chocolatey Blast crackers*, and *Kid Cuisine Magical Cheese Stuffed Crust Cheese Pizza* meals all met the criteria of the Smart Choices Program.

* When I asked Geoffrey Bible, former CEO of Philip Morris, about this shift toward more salt, sugar and fat in meals for kids, he smiled and noted that even in its earliest incarnation, Lunchables was held up for criticism. One article said something like, "If you take Lunchables apart, the healthiest item in it is the napkin."

~ Michael Moss, The Extraordinary Science of Junk Food

Worried About Your Cholesterol?

No problem. Just follow the Smart Choices Program, and you need worry no more. Eggs can't earn the coveted "Checkmark" because they have too much cholesterol. But if eggs are too rich, you can try some Hellman's mayonnaise or a low-fat Fudgsicle ... two more Smart Choices! (25)

Not surprisingly, there were critics ...

In response to critics, Michael Hughes, vice president for science and public policy at the *Keystone Center* and a member of the Smart Choices board, noted that none of the critics had presented scientific evidence that the program's criteria were out of line with a nutritious diet.

Besides Hughes argued, the directors carefully considered consumers' desires for taste, nutrition and convenience. "Sure, it might be ideal for growing arugula, pick it in the evening and make a big salad for dinner, but "that's not a choice everyone will make," he said.

Eileen T. Kennedy, president of the Smart Choices board and the dean of the *Friedman School of Nutrition Science and Policy at Tufts University*, said the program's criteria were based on government dietary guidelines and widely accepted nutritional standards.

"The *Checkmark* means the food item is a 'better for you' product, as opposed to having an x on it saying 'Don't eat this,'" Dr. Kennedy said. "Consumers are smart enough to deduce that if it doesn't have the *Checkmark* by implication, it's not a 'better-for-you' product.

Dr. Kennedy defended the products endorsed by the program, including sweet cereals. She said Froot Loops was better than other things parents could choose for their children. "You're rushing around, you're trying to think about healthy eating for your kids, and you have a choice between a doughnut and a cereal," Dr. Kennedy said, evoking a hypothetical parent in the supermarket. "So Froot Loops is a better choice."

(You can't make this up!)

Celeste Clark, a senior vice president at Kellogg's and a member of the Smart Choices board, put it another way:

OBESITY... *It's NOT what YOU THINK it is!*

"Froot Loops is an excellent source of many essential vitamins and minerals, and it is also a good source of fibre with only 12 grams of sugar. Small amounts of sugar added to nutrient-dense foods like breakfast cereals can make them taste better. That, in theory, will encourage people to eat more of them, which would increase the nutrients in their diet." (26)

We Don't Recommend ALL Junk Food, Just the "Healthiest" Junk Food

Michael Jacobson, executive director of the *Center for Science in the Public Interest*, an advocacy group, was part of a panel that helped devise the Smart Choices nutritional criteria – until he quit the previous September. He said the panel was dominated by members of the food industry, which skewed its decisions.

"It was paid for by the industry, and when industry put down its foot and said this is what we're doing, that was it, end of the story," he said. However, Dr. Kennedy and Dr. Clark, who were both on the panel, said industry members had not controlled the results. Hmmm ... who to believe?

In the end, just about all of Kellogg's cereals made the grade – in part because some were reformulated, which Dr. Clark called an added benefit of the program. Froot Loops, for example, has 3 grams less sugar per serving than it did *before* Smart Choices and 2 grams more fibre. (27)

See how easy it is to make "smart" choices and be healthy? All you gotta do is believe!

R.I.P. By October 2009, Smart Choices Program was pronounced dead.

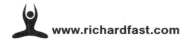

Coca-Cola Employs the Best "Scientific" Studies Money Can Buy!

Coca-Cola Activates "The Playbook"

→ Emphasize physical activity over diet. *Check.*

→ Criticize studies that hurt the industry as "junk science." *Check.*

→ State there are no good or bad foods; hence no food or food type (soft drinks, fast foods, etc.) should be targeted for change. *Double-check.*

→ Appear to be a socially responsible corporate citizen. *Check.*

→ Plant doubt when concerns are raised about the industry by funding research to produce desired results. *Check to the power of ten!*

In 2012, Coca-Cola's vice president and chief scientific officer, Rhona Applebaum, announced a major research effort to counter-evidence linking sodas to poor diets and health.

Company-funded research, she said, was essential to rebut the "agenda-driven science" of advocates for soda taxes. Coca-Cola intended to train journalists and engage scientists as partners to conduct both "defensive and offensive research." Otherwise, the industry would be at the mercy of "activists and crusading journalists." (29)

She wasn't kidding.

From 2008 to 2016, Coca-Cola funded studies and published 398 articles in 169 journals. The studies and resulting articles repeatedly found that physical activity is more effective than diet in weight control; sugars and soft drinks are harmless. (30)

Although there is a preponderance of research that underscores exercise as a markedly *inefficient* method for weight loss, that "minor" detail was not about to dissuade Coca-Cola from its mission.

Scientific Studies that Disprove Scientific Studies!

According to the Playbook, if you don't like the existing studies, don't panic; the company's "cheque-book" has an uncanny ability to produce "scientific" studies that will align with *any* interest.

To that end, Coca-Cola was in full support of a new "science-based" solution to the obesity crisis:

To maintain a healthy weight, get more exercise and worry less about cutting calories.

As it happens, a group of influential scientists were opposed to "conventional" science that found diet to be the primary cause of obesity. In response, they formed a non-profit organization called the *Global Energy Balance Network* (GEBN). This newly assembled group promoted the argument that weight-conscious Americans are overly fixated on how much they eat and drink while failing to pay enough attention to exercise.

"Most of the focus in the popular media and in the scientific press is, 'Oh they're eating too much, eating too much, eating too much' — blaming fast food, blaming sugary drinks and so on," the group's vice president, Steven N. Blair, an exercise scientist, says in a recent video announcing the new organization. "And there's really virtually no compelling evidence that that, in fact, is the cause." (31)

Health experts responded. This message is misleading and part of an effort by Coke to deflect criticism about the role sugary drinks have played in the spread of obesity and Type 2 diabetes. Coca-Cola uses the GEBN to convince the

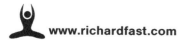

public that physical activity can offset a bad diet despite evidence that exercise has only a minimal impact on weight compared with what people consume. (32)

Coca-Cola Gets Caught with Its Hand in the "Selective-Science" Cookie Jar

A prominent piece published in the *New York Times* found that Coca-Cola had provided close to $4 million in funding for various research projects to two of the GEBN's founding members; Dr. Steven Blair, a professor at the *University of South Carolina* and Dr. Gregory Hand, dean of the *West Virginia University School of Public Health*. (29)

Records showed that GEBN's website, gebn.org, is registered to Coca-Cola headquarters in Atlanta, and the company is also listed as the site's administrator. GEBN's president, James Hill, a professor at the University of Colorado School of Medicine, said Coke had registered the website because the network's members did not know-how.

"They're not running the show," Hill said.
"We're running the show."

It's difficult to get a man to understand something when his salary depends on his not understanding it.
~ Upton Sinclair

When it was pointed out that GEBN's website failed to mention that Coke was funding their organization, Dr. Blair said this was an oversight that had been corrected. "As soon as we discovered that we didn't have not only Coca-Cola but other funding sources on the website, we put it on there," Dr. Blair said. "Does that make us totally corrupt in everything we do?"

Not to be dissuaded, the GEBN's website promises to be "the voice of science" in discussions about healthy lifestyle

OBESITY *It's NOT what YOU THINK it is!*

and contends that the concept of energy balance provides "a new science-based framework" for achieving a stable body weight. The group claims there is "strong evidence" that the key to preventing weight gain is not reducing food intake – as many public health experts recommend – but maintaining an active lifestyle and eating more calories.

"The media tends to blame the obesity pandemic on our poor eating habits," one news release stated. "But are those French fries really the culprit?" Dr. Blair advises, "you shouldn't believe everything you see on TV."

In recent years, Coke has donated money to build fitness centers in more than 100 schools across the country. It sponsors a program called *"Exercise is Medicine"* to encourage doctors to prescribe physical activity to patients.

And when Chicago's City Council proposed a soda tax in 2012 to help address the city's obesity problem, Coca-Cola donated $3 million to establish fitness programs in more than 60 of the city's community centers.

The initiative to tax soda ultimately failed.

"Reversing the obesity trend won't happen overnight," Coca-Cola said in an ad for its Chicago exercising initiative. "But for thousands of families in Chicago, it starts now, with the next push-up, a single sit-up or a jumping jack.

Coke Promises to Come Clean

The *New York Times* article, *"Coca-Cola Funds Scientists Who Shift Blame for Obesity Away from Bad Diets"* left many people concerned with obesity incredulous. (31)

Connecticut Representative Rosa DeLauro issued a statement: *"This research is reminiscent of the research conducted by the tobacco companies to mislead the public about the health risks of smoking. ... This new group and their*

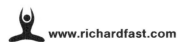

research are a sham. ... People want to be healthy, and they want their kids to be healthy and realize that drinks full of empty calories are not good for them." (32)

Shortly after, Coca-Cola's CEO, Muhtar Kent, submitted an op-ed piece for the *Wall Street Journal*, which said;

> "... I know our company can do a better job engaging both the public-health and scientific communities – and we will. ... in the future, we will act with even more transparency as we refocus our investments and our efforts on well-being. *(33)*

True to his word, Coca-Cola's website posted lists of its community and research partnerships for the past five years, and the lists would be updated regularly. The company revealed the names of the hundreds of individual health professionals, scientific experts, and organizations it had funded in the United States since 2010, along with the amounts it paid them. The funding totaled $21.8 million for research and $96.9 million for community partnerships. (34)

The site revealed that from 2010 to 2015, Coca-Cola had contributed $700,000 to the Academy of Nutrition and Dietetics, $2.9 million to the American Academy of Pediatrics, and $3.5 million to the American Academy of Family Physicians.

Within a week, Coca-Cola had ended its partnerships with these academies. By early November, the University of Colorado had returned Coke's $1 million grant given to Dr. Hill. The GEBN disbanded a week later. (34)

OBESITY *It's NOT what YOU THINK it is!*

How to Get a Planet Fat:
Create Food Addictions ... One Door at a Time

In 2017, the *New York Times* began publishing a series of investigative reports collectively titled "Planet Fat." The articles in this series explored the causes and the consequences of rising obesity rates around the world.

A particularly illuminating article titled *"How Big Business Got Brazil Hooked on Junk Food"* shows how the aggressive expansion of Western food companies into developing countries invariably *precedes* soaring rates of obesity.

Do you remember the fund-raiser drives your school held each year, just before Thanksgiving?

In my school, we all assembled in the auditorium, where the school principal got us all excited about selling chocolate bars to raise money for school trips, sports equipment, and entertainment.

After we were duly primed, a representative from the chocolate company got on stage to pitch us on the finer points of selling, while we dove after the chocolate samples he periodically lobbed into the audience. Each kid was issued a box of bars with promised incentives for the highest sales. Many of us begged for two boxes just to start.

For the chocolate companies, it was sales perfection. It didn't cost a dime in advertising, and what parent, aunt or uncle could refuse handing over a buck or two for such a worthy cause?

Brazil Gets Hooked

As sales growth began to slow in the wealthiest countries, multinational food companies like Nestlé, PepsiCo and General Mills turned their attention to developing nations.

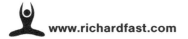

For Nestlé, the world's largest packaged food conglomerate, the goal for total global expansion was simple; get people to change from traditional diets to a Western-style diet of sugary drinks and ultra-processed food.

Since traditional advertising and distribution wouldn't work in the isolated pockets of Brazil, Nestlé duplicated the same technique that worked so beautifully for the chocolate industry in the North American school system; create an army of door-to-door vendors to penetrate households in Brazil's remotest corners.

Nestlés' Vendors

Nestlé began its door-to-door program in Brazil in 2007. Nestlés' website reports the program has grown to serve over 700,000 "low-income consumers each month.

According to Filipe Barbosa, a company supervisor, despite the country's continuing economic crisis, the vendor program has been growing 10 percent a year.

Sagging incomes among poor and working-class Brazilians had been a boon for direct sales. That's because Nestlé gives customers an entire month to pay for their purchases. It also helps that saleswomen – the program employs only women – know when their customers receive *Bolsa Famíla,* a monthly government subsidy for low-income households.

According to Barbosa, "the essence of our program is to reach the poor. What makes it work is the personal connection between the vendor and the customer."

Nestlés' program expansion provides economic benefits to people up and down the ladder, employing 21,000 people in Brazil. Since 2015 its apprenticeship program has trained over 7,000 people under the age of 30.

One of those trained vendors is Mrs. da Silva, who makes

OBESITY... *It's NOT what YOU THINK it is!*

$185 a month selling Nestlé products to customers in Fortaleza's slums who don't have ready access to a supermarket. She has high praise for the product she sells, exulting in the nutritional claims on the labels that boast of added vitamins and minerals.

"Everyone here knows that Nestlé products are good for you," she said, gesturing to cans of Mucilon, the infant cereal whose label says it is 'packed with calcium and niacin.'

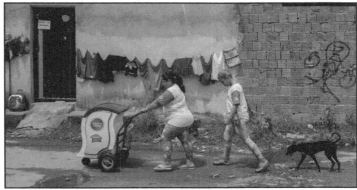

Nestlé vendors delivering food in the Fortaleza's slums. (35)

Nestlé portrays itself as a leader in its commitment to community and health. Two decades ago, it anointed itself a "nutrition health and wellness company."

"I'm a big believer in what we do at Nestlé," says Sean Westcott, Head of Global Products and Technology at Nestlé. "We use science and technology to enhance nature, not to replace nature."

"We're in this almost Utopian period where food is abundant. It's cheap. We solved the problem of food security. But in doing that, we didn't anticipate what the impact would be. Now we focus on things like reducing salt and reducing saturated fat. Over the years, we have reformulated nearly 9,000 products and delivered billions of servings fortified with vitamins and minerals."

~ Sean Westcott, Nestlé

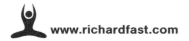

But of the 800 products that Nestlé says are available through its vendors, Mrs. da Silva says her customers are mostly interested in only about two dozen of them, virtually all sugar-sweetened items like *Kit-Kats, Nestlé Greek Red Berry*, a 3.5-ounce cup of yogurt with 17 grams of sugar; and *Chandelle Pacoca*, a peanut-flavored pudding in a container the same size as the yogurt that has 20 grams of sugar — nearly the entire World Health Organization's recommended daily limit.

Over Fed and Under Nourished

More than 1,000 miles south of Fortaleza, the effects of changing eating habits are evident at a brightly painted daycare center in São Paulo, Brazil's largest city.

When the daycare center was started in the early 1990s, the program, run by a Brazilian nonprofit group, had a straightforward mission: to alleviate under-nutrition among children who were not getting enough to eat in the city's most impoverished neighborhoods.

These days, many of those who attend are noticeably pudgy. The staff nutritionists note that some are worryingly short for their age due to diets heavy in salt, fat and sugar but lacking in the nourishment needed for healthy development.

The program, run by the *Center for Nutritional Recovery and Education*, includes pre-diabetic 10-year-olds with dangerously fatty livers, adolescents with hypertension and toddlers so poorly nourished they have trouble walking.

The rising obesity rates are largely associated with improved economics, as families with increasing incomes embrace the convenience, status and flavors offered by packaged foods.

Busy parents ply their toddlers with instant noodles and

OBESITY *It's NOT what YOU THINK it is!*

frozen chicken nuggets, meals that are often accompanied by soda. Studies have found that rice, beans, salad, and grilled meats — building blocks of the traditional Brazilian diet — are falling by the wayside.

Profits are Booming ... All is Well

Public health advocates have criticized Nestlé for its door-to-door marketing as an insidious campaign to reach every doorstep in its effort to become central to communities in the developing world.

Industry defenders say that **processed foods*** are essential to feed a growing, urbanizing world of people, many of them with rising incomes, demanding convenience. CEO Mark Schneider told investors that developing markets now provide Nestlé with 42 percent of its sales.

*Please Note: Be particularly mindful of the interchangeable <u>misuse</u> of the terms "processed-food" and "ultra-processed-food." ALL food is processed to some degree. Ultra-processed food is <u>NOT</u> food.

"We're not going to get rid of all factories and go back to growing all-grain. It's nonsense. It's not going to work," said Mike Gibney, a professor emeritus of food and health at University College Dublin and a consultant to Nestlé. If I ask 100 Brazilian families to stop eating **processed food,*** I have to ask myself: What will they eat? Who will feed them? How much will it cost?

"What we have is a war between two food systems, a traditional diet of *real food* once produced by the farmers around you and the producers of **ultra-processed food** designed to be over-consumed and which, in some cases are addictive," said Carlos Monteiro, a professor of nutrition and public health at the University of São Paulo.

"It's a war," he said, "but one food system has disproportionately more power than the other." (35)

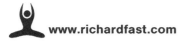

Malaysia Drinks Industry Kool-Aid, Becoming the Fattest Nation in Asia

In *New York Times'* continuing *"Planet Fat"* series is another jaw-dropping example of the outright duplicity between Big Food and so-called "nutritional" studies.

In the *New York Times'* piece titled *"In Asia's Fattest Country, Nutritionists Take Money from Food Giants,"* the graft is so transparent it would make La Cosa Nostra blush.

It's no secret that Big Food companies "invest" heavily in support of their local nutrition scientists through sponsorship of research projects, scholarships, consulting fees and nutrition conferences; one of the more striking examples of the shared interests between Big Food and "science" is Malaysia's Dr. Tee E Siong, the country's leading nutrition expert.

As head of the *Nutrition Society of Malaysia*, Dr. Tee produced several articles for peer-reviewed academic journals.

Among his published works was a study concluding that children who drank malted breakfast beverages (a category dominated in Malaysia by Milo, a sugary powder drink made by Nestlé) were more likely to be physically active and spend less time in front of a computer or television. (36)

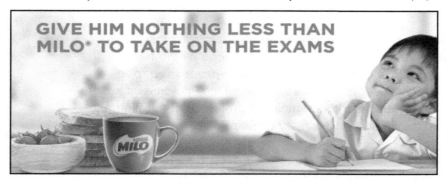

GIVE HIM NOTHING LESS THAN MILO® TO TAKE ON THE EXAMS

OBESITY *It's NOT what YOU THINK it is!*

Scientists weren't the only ones vetting the material. According to the terms of their sponsorship, Nestlé gets to read the papers *before* publication as part of a written agreement with Dr. Tee's *Nutrition Society*. As Nestlé phrased it, their review of the malted breakfast study was merely to "ensure that the methodology was scientifically correct."

In addition to sponsorship from Nestlé, Dr. Tee's work has been funded by Kellogg's, PepsiCo, and Tate & Lyle, one of the world's biggest makers of high-fructose corn syrup. He said scientists need cooperation and financial support from companies, who can supply much-needed resources.

Dr. Tee points out that traditional Malaysian cuisine — curries and other sugar-laden street foods — are key contributors to obesity but noted that working with street vendors and mom-and-pop companies to make their food healthier is difficult. Working with multinational companies is easier and more productive, he said.

Smart Choices Labeling ... Déjà vu All Over Again?

The ethos of corporate partnership runs through several health initiatives in Malaysia. A Health Ministry committee teamed up with the *Federation of Malaysian Manufacturers*, which includes representatives of major food companies, to develop a labeling system for the public. The labels tell consumers which packaged foods are a "healthier choice" than others in the same category. (37)

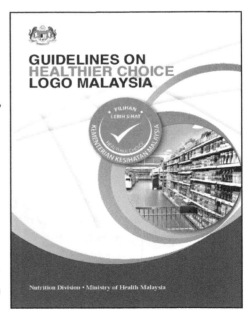

Malaysian supermarkets are loaded with products now found across the globe: instant noodles, spaghetti sauce, soda, and rows of sugary cereals, including Nestlé's *Stars*, which is 28 percent sugar and has a bright red circle on the bottom

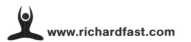

right of the box that says, "Selected Healthier Choice Malaysia Ministry of Health."

In 2014, Dr. Tee created the Southeast Asian Public Health Nutrition Network, or SEA-PHN, with nutrition leaders from Thailand, Indonesia, the Philippines, and Vietnam. Much of the network's funding comes from Danone, Nestlé, PepsiCo and other large food companies, whose logos are displayed prominently on the SEA-PHN website and its annual reports.

Dr. Tee says nearly all the group's funding comes from corporate sponsorship and fees for attending conferences.

We have to stop blaming the multinationals. The real problem isn't the type of food people eat, but how much of it and their lifestyle. Malaysians are always eating. They don't exercise. But you don't need to go to the gym. You need to walk outside. It's free. Get off your chair and move!"

~ Dr. Tee E Siong

For his part, Dr. Tee said the obesity risk in Malaysia would be worse without companies' help, and he couldn't accomplish his goals without their support.

"There are some people who say that we should not accept money for projects, for research studies. I'm aware of that," Dr. Tee said. "I have two choices: Either I don't do anything, or I work with companies."

The Value of Dr. Tee's "Work" Speaks for Itself

In 2019, the National Health and Morbidity survey revealed that 50.1 percent of Malaysian's adults were obese or overweight. Malaysia – being the fattest country in Asia notwithstanding – also has the second-highest child obesity rate in children aged five to 19. (37, 38)

The Takeaway

The Big Food companies have one mandate; maximize profit at all costs; like the scorpion, it's just their nature.

Unfortunately, their highest profit margins come from designing and selling the cheapest ultra-processed foods. These "so-called" foods are easy to produce, highly addictive, and since they're stripped of nutrients, they guarantee overindulgence.

As we will see in the next part *(The Cause),* ultra-processed foods are directly, and almost inclusively responsible for our declining health and rising obesity.

What I found, over four years of research and reporting, was a conscious effort — taking place in labs and marketing meetings and grocery store aisles — to get people hooked on foods that are convenient and inexpensive.

~ Michael Moss (39)

The Dilemma

It's in the Big Food companies' best interest to sell as much ultra-processed food as possible. It's in our best interest to eliminate it as much as possible.

A War of Conflicting Interests

As we have seen, we cannot rely on businesses, government legislation or scientific bodies to right this listing ship-of-health. Our health is on each of us. We need to take what's being done to our children and us as a personal affront. We're being conned, and addicted by Big Food's advertising and food manipulation.

Big Food rakes in billions of dollars while it systematically makes us sick and obese, and the reality is ... they could care less.

That should piss us off enough to fight back! After all, what's at stake is nothing less than our health and the future health of our children.

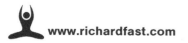

References

1. Biakolo, K., "A Brief History of the TV Dinner," Smithsonian Magazine, Arts & Culture, November, 2020

2. Kessler, D., "The End of Overeating: Taking Control of the Insatiable American Appetite," Rodale Inc. New York, NY, 2009

3. Friedman, M., Capitalism and Freedom, 40th Anniversary Edition, University of Chicago Press, Ltd. Chicago, IL. 60637, 2020

4. Michele Simon, "Appetite for Profit: How the Food Industry Undermines our Health and How to Fight Back," Nation Books, 1290 Avenue of the Americas, New York, N.Y., 2006

5. Malik, R., "Catch Me If You Can: Big Food Using Big Tobacco's Playbook? Applying the Lessons from Big Tobacco to Attack the Obesity Epidemic," Harvard Library, December, 6, 2010

6. Cummings, K. M., Morley, C.P., Hyland, A., "Failed Promises of the Cigarette Industry and Its Effect on Consumer Misperceptions About the Health Risks of Smoking," Tobacco Control 2002;11(Suppl I):110–i117

7. Kessler, D., "A Question of Intent: A Great American Battle with a Deadly Industry," Public Affairs, Perseus Books, New York, NY 10107, 2001

8. Brownell, K., Warner, K. E., "The Perils of Ignoring History: Big Tobacco Played Dirty and Millions Died. How Similar is Big Food?" The Milbank Quarterly, 2009 Mar; 87(1):259-294

9. Michaels, D., "Doubt Is Their Product: How Industry's Assault on Science Threatens Your Health," New York: Oxford University Press; 2008

10. Mooney, C., "Republican War on Science," New York: Basic Books, 2006

11. RJR Nabisco. Winston-Salem, N.C.: 1996. Annual Meeting of Shareholders (proceedings) pp.61-62 April 17

12. Holguin, J., "Battle of the Widening Bulge: Lawyers Who Battled Big Tobacco Size Up Fast Food Industry," CBC Evening News, Aug. 8, 2002

13. Brown & Williamson. Implications of Battelle Hippo I & II and the Griffith Filter (memo marked "Strictly Private and Confidential"), July 17. 1963. Available at http://legacy.library.ucsf.edu/tid/xrc72d00/pdf

14. Dunn, W. L. Jr., 1972 Philip Morris document. 1972. Available at http://legacy.library.ucsf.edu/action/document/page?tid=itb12a00

15. Hurt, R.D., Robertson, C.R., "Prying Open the Door to the Tobacco Industry's Secrets about Nicotine: The Minnesota Tobacco Trial," Journal of the American Medical Association 1998;280:1173–81.

16. Sebrie, E. M., Glantz, S. A., "Attempts to Undermine Tobacco Control: Tobacco Industry "Youth Smoking Prevention" Programs to Undermine Meaningful Tobacco Control in Latin America," American Journal of Public Health, 2007;97:1357-67

17. Wakefield, M., et al., "Effect of Televised, Tobacco Company-Funded Smoking Prevention Advertising on Youth Smoking-Related Beliefs, Intentions, and Behavior," American Journal of Public Health, 2006;96:2154-60

18. Sharma, L., Teret, S. T., Brownell, K. D., "The Food Industry and Self-Regulation: Standards to Promote Success and to Avoid Public Health Failures," American Journal of Public Health, Sept:20, 2011

19. Council of Better Business Bureaus. Press release: Better Business Bureau Announces Food and Beverage Advertising Commitments from 11 Industry Leaders, July 18, 2007

20. Advocacy Institute. "Smoke & Mirrors: How the Tobacco Industry Buys & Lies Its Way to Power & Profits," Washington D.C.: 1998

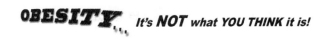
OBESITY It's NOT what YOU THINK it is!

21. Warner, K. E., "What's a Cigarette Company to Do?" American Journal of Public Health, 2002;92:897-900

22. Simon. M., "Nutrition Scientists on the Take from Big Food: Has the American Society for Nutrition Lost All Credibility?" Eat, Drink Politics, June 14, 2015

23. Simon, M., "And Now a Word From Our Sponsors: Are America's Nutrition Professionals in the Pocket of Big Food?," Eat Drink Politics, Jan 2013, www.eatdrinkpolitics.com/wp-content/uploads/AND_Corporate_Sponsorship

24. Lupton, J.R., Balentine, D.A., Black, R.M., et al., "The Smart Choices Front-of-Package Nutrition Labeling Program: Rationale and Development of the Nutrition Criteria," Am J Clin Nutr. 2010, 91(4):1078s–1089s

25. Wanjek, C., "New 'Smart Choices' Food Labels Are Deceptive," Live Science, Sept. 9, 2009

26. Neuman, W., "For Your Health, Froot Loops," The New York Times, Sept. 4, 2009

27. MacVean, M., "Smart Choice Food Label: A Sign of Nutrition or Marketing?", Los Angeles Times, Sept 29, 2009

28. Smart Choices Program, "Smart Choices Program™ Postpone Active Operations," press release, Oct 23, 2009

29. Applebaum, R.S., "Balancing the Debate," Presentation to The Food Industry: Trends & Opportunities, 29th International Sweetener Symposium, Coeur d'Alene, Idaho, Aug 7, 2012, www.phaionline.org/wp-content/uploads /2015/08/Rhona-Applebaum.pdf.

30. Serôdio, P.M., McKee, M., Stuckler, D., "Coca-Cola—a Model of Transparency in Research Partnerships? A Network Analysis of Coca-Cola's Research Funding (2008–2016)," Public Health Nutr. 2018, 21(9):1594–1607;

31. O'Connor, A., "Coca-Cola Funds Scientists Who Shift Blame for Obesity Away from Bad Diets," The New York Times, August 9, 2015

32. DeLauro, R., "DeLauro statement on Coca-Cola Funding Biased Obesity Research," press release, DeLauro.House.gov, Aug 10, 2015

33. Kent, M., "Coca-Cola: We'll Do Better," Wall Street J., Aug 19, 2015

34. Douglas, S., "Our Commitment to Transparency: Our Actions and Way Forward," Coca-Cola Journey, Sep 22, 2015

35. Jacobs, A., Richtel, M., "How Big Business Got Brazil Hooked on Junk Food," New York Times, Sept. 16, 2017

36. Mohamed, J., et al., "Characteristics Associated with the Consumption of Malted Drinks Among Malaysian Primary School Children: Findings from the MyBreakfast Study," BMC Public Health, Dec. 2015; 15:1322

37. Fuller, T., O"Connor, A., Richtel, M., "In Asia's Fattest Country, Nutritionists Take Money From Food Giants," New York Times, Dec. 23, 2017

38. Chalil, M., "Cling on to Traditional Food Culture to Address Fattest Nation Reputation, UK Expert Advises Malaysians," Yahoo! News, Aug 5, 2021

39. Moss, M., "The Extraordinary Science of Addictive Junk Food,: The New York Times Magazine, Feb. 20, 2013

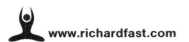

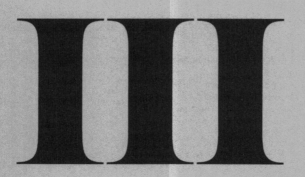

part III

The Cause

Cause ~ *The source of, or reason for, an event or action; that which produces or effects a result.*
Merriam-Webster

Is Global Obesity the Result of a Single Cause?

The truth is, the *cause* of "one's" obesity is far more complex than a simple physics equation such as; *too many calories in ... not enough calories burned.* Obesity invariably results from a combination of economics, social science, psychology, biology, nutrition, endocrinology, willpower, habit and just about anything else we want to throw in the mix. In other words, the factors that drive *one's* obesity are as myriad as the number of people who suffer from it.

However, to conclude that the rapid rise in *global* obesity is too vast and complex to corral into a singular cause fails to address several overarching questions such as:

- How is it that people who were overweight stood out from the general population for thousands of years?
- Why did obesity suddenly begin in the mid-70s in the USA and indiscriminately affect millions of people? (1)
- Although the speed and extent of weight gain varied somewhat by age, gender, and ethnicity, why did all subgroups become heavier at the same time? (2)
- While, on average, all Americans were getting heavier since the mid-80s, why were the heaviest people gaining disproportionately more weight than the others?

To answer the above, the question isn't what causes obesity. Instead, the question to ask and answer is; **what *singular* factor could cause indiscriminate, population-wide obesity across the entire planet?**

The short answer is the one thing we all have in common; food. The expanded answer is the rapid increase in food production that led to a cascade of results. For example, greater production increased portion sizes, accelerated marketing, availability, affordability, cultural shifts, fast-food outlets and the widespread introduction of cheap and potent sweetening agents, such as high-fructose corn syrup, which infiltrated the food system and affected the whole population simultaneously. [3, 4]

When we track the rising obesity rates anywhere on the planet, invariably, the "smoking gun" is always the same ... ultra-processed food.

The Birth of Ultra-Processed Food and the Simultaneous Rise in Obesity

For the past 50 years, we've been told that saturated fats, the kind you find in some oils, meat, and dairy, were the number one cause of heart disease. So, when Big Food were told to trim the fat, they were happy to oblige. They made a fortune manufacturing low-fat products, which they promised would make people live longer and healthier. As it turned out, the exact opposite occurred. In trimming the fat, they had to figure out how to replace the taste and texture of fatty food, and all it required was a little chemistry and a lot of extra sugar.

In fact, more than half the calories we consume come from food that isn't food; they're ultra-processed concoctions that contain starch, sugar, salt, hydrogenated oils, preservatives, and additives, lots of additives.

Compared to real food, they have three times the amount of free sugar, twice as much sodium, far more calories and little fibre, minerals and vitamins.

Ultra-processed foods now make up more than half of the calories consumed in the UK, US, and Canada, and the rest of the world is rapidly catching up.

Brazil's Obesity Detective Identifies the Killer

Carlos Monteiro got his start in medicine in the 1970s as a pediatrician working in poor villages and slums in the state of São Paulo, Brazil. Back then, his patients were hungry. Many were frail, underweight, and stunted.

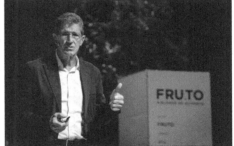

Today he's focused on the opposite problem: In the last decade, the country's obesity rate has nearly doubled to 20 percent, and the portion of overweight people has almost tripled to 58 percent.

Dr Carlos Monteiro. Professor of Nutrition and Public Health at the University of Sao Paulo, Brazil and Head of the University's Centre for Epidemiological Studies in Health and Nutrition.

In the early years of this millennium, Monteiro noticed a paradox. The data showed people were consuming fewer beans, rice, milk, eggs, and produce. Sales of table sugar and soy oil were going down. Still, the rates of obesity and type 2 diabetes were going up.

Having tracked the nation's diet for many years, in 2003, Monteiro named *the cause* of Brazil's soaring obesity problem; ultra-processed products. The traditional Brazilian diet of rice and beans was being replaced by a food system controlled by transnational corporations.

To Monteiro, the problem was so obvious it no longer made sense to talk in terms of food groups and nutrients. A more meaningful distinction was to focus on how the food is produced.

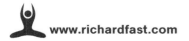

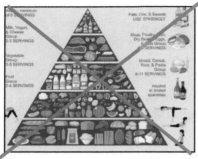

"The traditional food pyramids and recommendations are based on the assumption that people still cook from scratch."
~ Carlos Monteiro

Recognizing the country's soaring obesity rates, the Health Ministry contracted Monteiro and a team of Brazilian nutritionists to write a *practical* food guide related to how Brazilians live.

As Monteiro said, "People don't need to understand the difference between saturated fats and unsaturated fats, and we don't think normal people will decide what to eat based on nutrients." (5)

The Brazilian Food Guide was born.

Brazil Introduces a "Practical" and Revolutionary Food Guide

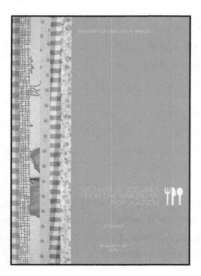

In 2014 Brazil introduced a food guide that shocked the world. Not only was it radically different from any other food guide ever issued, but it got rave reviews from North America's harshest nutrition critics. (6)

What made it so unique was its complete avoidance of plotting foods into pyramids and plates. It contained no information on calories or serving sizes, nor did it suggest percentages of fats, proteins or carbohydrates. Neither did it dwell on nutrients, calories or weight loss.

Instead, it addressed lifestyle and the importance of sharing, eating together, learning

OBESITY *It's NOT what YOU THINK it is!*

to cook and getting pleasure from food.

What's so refreshing about this guide is the message that you should not necessarily avoid ingredients such as cooking oil and sugar, because these are essential for many aspects of cooking. The guidelines carry a rare understanding that culinary tradition is an integral part of our culture and identity and an important link to previous generations. In this way, food can help us find meaning in our lives, increase social cohesion, and connect us to our past.

> *In epidemiology, we see the vector of a disease. So, mosquitoes are the vector of malaria. The vector of obesity is ultra-processed foods. Obesity is increasing all over the world. In Brazil, every year, we have one million new cases of obesity.*
>
> *~ Carlos Monteiro*

These benefits are increasingly shown to have profound implications for both mental and physical wellbeing.

The overarching message of the Brazilian food guide was to stress that eating healthy came down to the degree that one avoided eating ultra-processed foods.

"Processed" Food Is a Critical Component to Our Health

For most of our history, our ancestors would have experienced hunger far more than satiety. For hunter-gatherers, preserving calories could be the difference between life and death during the inevitable lean times.

To that end, we learned how to process and preserve food, which has been a critical component of our survival. We salt and smoke meats to ensure that microorganisms that attempt to steal them will die of dehydration. We pasteurize and freeze perishable vegetables to kill the microbes already on them and to exclude all newcomers. We make fruit preserves with high concentrations of sugar for much the same reason.

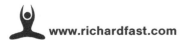

The NOVA Classification of Processed Food

The *Brazilian Food Guide* and the NOVA classification divided food into four groups to clear up the confusion caused by the fact that, previously, "processed" meant different things to different people.

NOVA GROUP 1 Minimally Processed & Natural Foods	The first category is natural or minimally processed foods. Natural foods are those obtained directly from plants or animals (such as green leaves and fruits, or eggs and milk) and purchased for consumption without undergoing alteration following their removal from nature. Minimally processed foods have had some minor cosmetic things done to them, such as removing inedible or unwanted parts. Freezing, boiling, canning, vacuum packing, and pasteurization are also considered minimal processing.
NOVA GROUP 2 Processed Culinary Ingredients	These are products extracted from natural foods or from nature itself and used for seasoning and cooking food to create culinary preparations. Pressed vegetable oils, butter, sugar and molasses obtained from cane or beet; honey extracted from combs and syrup from maple trees, salt, corn starch
NOVA GROUP 3 Processed Foods	This category consists of products that are manufactured with the addition of salt or sugar to natural or minimally processed foods. Examples include canned and bottled vegetables or fruits, cheeses, and breads. Here the object of processing the food is "to increase the durability of group 1 foods, or to modify or enhance their sensory qualities."

OBESITY... *It's NOT what YOU THINK it is!*

The Unsavoury Truth of Ultra-Processed "Food"

As noted in the previous part (*The Culprit*), the terms "processed food" and "ultra-processed food" are often used interchangeably by the Food Industry to sow confusion and doubt. But let's be clear; Ultra-processed foods (UPFs) are formulations of ingredients, mostly of exclusive industrial use, that result from a series of industrial processes (hence ultra-processed).

Processes enabling the manufacture of UPF involve several steps and different industries. It starts with *fractioning* whole foods into substances that include sugars, oils and fats, proteins, starches, and fibre. These substances are often obtained from a few high-yield plant foods (corn, wheat, soy, cane or beet) and from puréeing or grinding animal carcasses, usually from intensive livestock farming. (8)

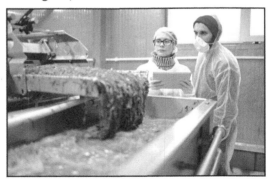

Food substances of no or rare culinary use, and used only in the manufacture of ultra-processed foods, include varieties of sugars (fructose, high-fructose corn syrup, 'fruit juice concentrates,' invert sugar, maltodextrin, dextrose, lactose), modified oils (hydrogenated oils) and protein sources (hydrolyzed proteins, soy protein isolate, gluten, casein, whey protein and 'mechanically separated meat').

Cosmetic additives are flavours, flavour enhancers, colours, emulsifiers*, emulsifying salts, sweeteners, thickeners, anti-foaming, bulking, carbonating, foaming, gelling, and glazing agents. These additives disguise undesirable sensory properties created by ingredients or processes. (8)

* The Hidden Danger of Ultra-Processed Food

In a way, ultra-processed foods result from advances in food science and food technology. But it is not an advance in human health because our bodies aren't prepared to be fed with these formulations because they lack the food matrix.

For instance, when these formulations-combine sugar, salt, fats and additive flavours, you get products that tend to be consumed in excess. These formulations fool our bodies into consuming more than we need.

* Emulsifiers are very common in ultra-processed foods. But they're problematic because they can affect the impermeability of our intestinal cells, which short-circuits our body's natural ability to resist the absorption of specific molecules. That's why we see in epidemiological studies that the more ultra-processed food a person consumes, the higher the risk of several chronic diseases, including obesity, cardiovascular diseases and certain types of cancer. (9)

OBESITY *It's NOT what YOU THINK it is!*

UPFs: Tasty, Cheap, Ubiquitous and Oh So Profitable

Processes and ingredients used to manufacture UPFs are designed to create highly profitable products (low-cost ingredients, long shelf-life, branded products), which are liable to displace all other NOVA food groups. (8)

Marketing strategies used worldwide by transnational corporations include vivid packaging, health claims, special deals with retailers to secure prime shelf space, the establishment of franchised catering outlets, and campaigns using social, electronic, broadcast and print media, including to children and in schools, often with vast budgets. All this explains why ultra-processed foods have *"successfully"* displaced "unprocessed" or minimally processed foods in most parts of the world. (10)

To be clear, consumed in isolation and moderation, ultra-processed foods are not dangerous because their long shelf life makes them micro-biologically safe.

However, what happens to our bodies when nearly 70 percent (11) of our diet is made up of ultra-processed foods?

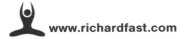

Why Are Ultra-Processed Foods SO Hard to Resist?

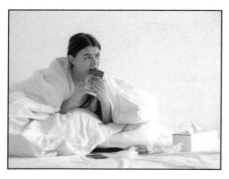

If you have a knee-bending weakness for certain foods, it's not because you're lacking control. There's a vast, underground industry dedicated to creating hyper-palatable foods that are so tasty they leave you practically powerless to resist.

My guess is that you've never found your hand at the bottom of a basket of apples after inexplicably gorging down the entire container. Why is that? Because the characteristics and properties of natural food are entirely different from those of ultra-processed food.

Understanding "Real" Food

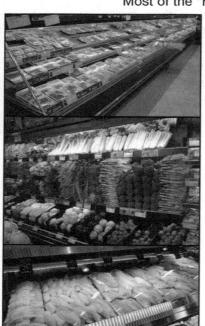

Most of the "real" food found in grocery stores, such as fresh produce, meats, and artisan cheese, is on the perimeter. These foods are easy to understand. They don't feel it's necessary to claim their goodness, ingredients, or percentage of fibre. To real food, these things are self-evident; they contain all that you need.

Food – roots, greens, lean meats – is generally fibrous and low in calories per serving. It requires an average of 25 chews per mouthful, which automatically makes you slow down. When that happens, your natural satiety signals can accurately gauge when you've had enough, which is why you don't habitually overeat fresh meat, vegetables, or fruit.

Real Food: *It's nutritious, satisfying, and healthy. That's all there is to know!*

OBESITY... *It's NOT what YOU THINK it is!*

Understanding Ultra-Processed Food

Ultra-processed foods (UPFs) insist on shouting their qualities; "we're high in fibre, we've added vitamins, we're organic, low-fat, 10% real fruit juice!"

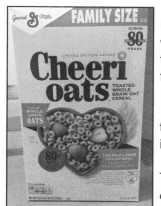

Ultra-processed food has its own language, which means you need to speak the lingo to "really" understand it. Ultra-processed food expresses itself in terms such as *'mouth feel,' 'maximum bite force,'* and *'sensory-specific satiety,* which means the rate at which a food product loses its appeal as its being eaten.

Then there are the terms like *'vanishing caloric density'*, which describes food that dissolves quickly in the mouth to trick the brain into believing that no calories have been ingested; thus no signals of satiety.

"If you're concerned about your health, you should probably avoid products that make health claims. Why? Because a health claim on a food product is a strong indication it's not really food, and food is what you want to eat"

~ Michael Pollan

Ultra-Processed Food is More Than a Language; It's a Complete Science!

New York Times investigative reporter Michael Moss spent four years sketching the secrets of the food industry's scientists.

"I was totally surprised," he said. "I spent time with the top scientists at the largest companies in this country, and it's amazing how much math and science and regression analysis and energy they put into finding the perfect amount of salt, sugar and fat that will send us over the moon and will send their products flying off the shelves and have us buy more, eat more and ...make more money for them." (12)

The "Holy Trinity" of Big Food

The common denominator among the most irresistible ultra-processed foods is salt, fat and refined carbohydrates, a potent combination rarely seen in naturally occurring

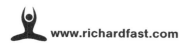

foods. Foods found in nature are rich in either fat or carbohydrates, but typically not both.

While the industry shuns the word "addiction" more than any other, the fact is their research has shown that when they hit the "right" amounts, we can't stop eating. It's called the *'bliss point'*, that perfect blend of salt, sugar and fat. (13)

When Moss began investigating the science of food processing, he said he was at first skeptical of the concept of food-addiction ... "Until I spent some time with the top scientists in the U.S. who say that 'yes, for some people, the most highly loaded salty, sugary, fatty foods are every bit as addictive as some narcotics.'" (14)

In some ways, of course, food is more insidious than drugs because there's no such thing as abstinence, no such thing as never starting in the first place, no such thing as being able to say, "Food? Never touch the stuff." You eat because you'll die if you don't, so you spend your life in a sort of nutritional two-step—a little but not too much; go overboard today, cut back tomorrow; eat the good stuff but never the junk. Sometimes you succeed at all of that, and other times you fail terribly; we all do. (15)

Are Ultra-Processed Foods Addictive?

Dr. Ashley Gearhardt is a clinical psychologist who helped develop the *Yale Food Addiction Scale*, a survey used to determine whether a person shows signs of addictive behaviour toward food.

In one study involving more than 500 people, Dr. Gearhardt and her colleagues found that certain foods were especially prone to elicit "addictive-like" eating behaviours; intense cravings, a loss of control, and an inability to cut back despite experiencing harmful consequences and a strong desire to stop eating them.

At the top of the list were pizza, chocolate, potato chips, cookies, ice cream, French fries, and cheeseburgers – no surprise there. However, like cigarettes and cocaine, processed foods share much in common with addictive substances. Their ingredients come from naturally occurring plants and foods that are stripped of components that slow their absorption, such as fibre, water, and protein. Then their most pleasurable ingredients are refined and processed into products that are rapidly absorbed into the bloodstream, enhancing their ability to light up regions of the brain that regulate reward, emotion, and motivation. (16)

As Dr. Gearhardt noted, "People don't experience an addictive behavioural response to naturally occurring foods that are good for our health, like strawberries. This subset of highly processed foods is engineered in a way that's so similar to how we create other addictive substances. These are the foods that can trigger a loss of control and compulsive, problematic behaviours that parallel what we see with alcohol and cigarettes." (17)

According to Bruce Bradley, a former food industry executive who spent 15 years working for some of the largest food corporations:

"These products are designed to keep you coming back to eat more and more and more. Ingredients are bundled under what may seem like relatively innocuous labels like 'natural flavours' or even 'artificial flavours' when truly they are much more surprising when consumers understand what it is.

We're not talking about food being real anymore. It's synthetic, completely contrived and created. There are so many problems about that because our bodies are tricked, and when our bodies are tricked repeatedly, dramatic things can happen, like weight gain, endocrine disruption, diabetes and hypertension." (12)

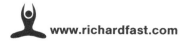 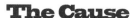

Ultra-Processed Food – Habit or Addiction?

Food companies vehemently deny any notion that ultra-processed food is addictive. However, many scientific studies would suggest just the opposite – thus, another rabbit hole in the nutritional field of endless argument and contradiction.

But here's the thing, whether ultra-processed food *is* or *isn't* addictive isn't the point (although the evidence strongly suggests it is), it *is* habit-forming, and habits are notoriously difficult to break.

It's safe to assume that science and Big Food will argue their positions for years to come ... meanwhile obesity and disease doggedly continues its relentless march across the globe.

Whenever ultra-processed food becomes a high percentage of a population's diet, obesity soars. The food industry argues that correlation does not equal causation. Until recently, they may have had a case, but as we will see in the three upcoming studies, ultra-processed food is unequivocally the primary cause of our obesity pandemic.

3 "Scientific" Studies Confirm Ultra-Processed Food Drives Obesity

What Would It Take to Change Your Mind?

In his thought-provoking book, *Mental Immunity*, author Andy Norman begins a section titled, *"What Would Change Your Mind?"*

He then tells a intriguing story that juxtaposes the difference between *"one's love for truth"* and one who *"tries to make true that which he loves"*.

In February 2014, two contestants entered a packed auditorium at the *Creation Museum* in Petersburg, Kentucky.

They were there to debate the scientific merits of the biblical account of Creation.

The pro-biblical debater, Ken Ham, was defending the literal truth of the origins story of Genesis. His opponent, science educator and TV personality Bill "the Science Guy" Nye, stated that the Genesis story was scientifically untenable.

Not surprisingly, neither man succeeded in persuading the other to change his mind, but what was fascinating was their answers to a question posed by the debate's moderator:

> "Gentlemen," he asked, "what would it take to change your mind?"

In context, he probably meant "change your mind about evolution," but his framing of the question was suggestively general.

Ham replied, "I'm a Christian. No one is ever going to convince me that the word of God is not true."

Nye responded with one word: "evidence." It was a perfect expression of the scientific attitude: Give me good evidence, and I'll change my mind.

Study #1

A "True" Scientist Changes His Mind

Evidence! Dr. Kevin Hall would accept nothing less.

The first time Hall heard anyone talk about ultra-processed food, he thought it was a "nonsense definition." It was 2016, and Hall – who studies how people put on weight at the *National Institute of Diabetes and Digestive and Kidney Diseases* at Bethesda, Maryland – was at a conference chatting with a representative from PepsiCo who scornfully mentioned the new Brazilian set of food guidelines and

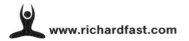

specifically the directive to avoid ultra-processed foods. Hall agreed that this was a silly rule because obesity had nothing to do with food processing as far as he was concerned. (12)

When Hall started to read through the scientific literature on ultra-processed foods, he noticed that all the damning evidence against them took the form of *correlation* rather than absolute proof. Most studies fell under the umbrella of epidemiology: the study of health patterns across populations – studies which Dr. Hall found less than convincing.

Just because people who eat a lot of ultra-processed foods are more likely to be obese or suffer from cancer does not mean that ultra-processed foods cause obesity and cancer. Correlation is not causation.

At the end of 2018, Hall and his colleagues became the first scientists to test – in randomized controlled conditions – whether diets high in ultra-processed foods could cause overeating and weight gain.

Researcher Finds the Evidence ... Surprising

Like many other scientists, Dr. Hall knew that people in lower socioeconomic brackets tend to consume the most ultra-processed foods. They also tend to smoke more, exercise less and engage in other unhealthy behaviours. As a result, large population studies cannot entirely separate the effects of eating ultra-processed foods from other lifestyle factors that influence obesity and disease.

To address this problem, Hall and his colleagues recruited 20 healthy men and women. The number of people in the study was necessarily small because the subjects had to spend 28 days living at the research facility (Metabolic Clinical Research Unit, National Institute of Health) eating only their prescribed diets.

OBESITY.., *It's NOT what YOU THINK it is!*

Dr. Hall's Study

→ Participants were ten male and ten female "weight-stable" adults whose average age was 31.

→ Subjects were randomly assigned to either the ultra-processed or unprocessed diet for two weeks, followed immediately by the alternate diet for the final two weeks.

→ During each diet phase, subjects were presented three meals daily and instructed to consume as much or as little as desired. Up to 60 minutes were allotted for each meal.

→ Menus rotated on a 7-day schedule, and the meals were designed to be well matched across diets for total calories, energy density, macronutrients, fibre, sugars, and sodium, but widely differing in the percentage of calories derived from *ultra-processed* versus *unprocessed* foods as defined according to the NOVA 4-group classification scheme.

→ The researchers prepared all their meals and snacks, tracked every morsel of food they ate, and carefully analyzed the effects of those foods on their weight, body fat, hormones, and other biomarkers. (18)

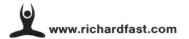

Day One: Processed Diet

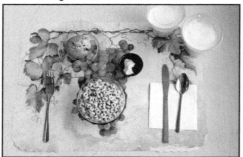

Breakfast: Honey Nut Cheerios (General Mills); whole milk with NutriSource fiber; blueberry muffin (Otis Spunkmeyer); margarine (Glenview Farms)

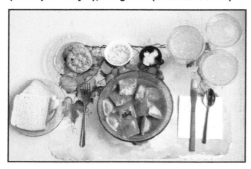

Lunch: Beef ravioli (Chef Boyardee); Parmesan cheese (Roseli); white bread (Ottenberg); margarine (Glenview Farms); diet lemonade (Crystal Light) with NutriSource fiber; oatmeal raisin cookies (Otis Spunkmeyer)

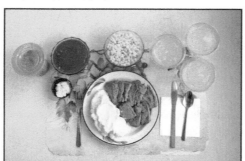

Dinner: Steak (Tyson); gravy (McCormick); mashed potatoes (Basic American Foods); margarine (Glenview Farms); corn (canned, Giant); diet lemonade (Crystal Light) with NutriSource fiber; low-fat chocolate milk (Nesquik) with NutriSource fiber

Day One: Whole Food Diet

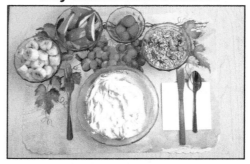

Breakfast: Greek yogurt (Fage) parfait with strawberries, bananas, walnuts (Diamond), salt and olive oil; apple slices with fresh squeezed lemon

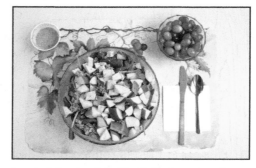

Lunch: Spinach salad with chicken breast, apple slices, bulgur (Bob's Red Mill), sunflower seeds and grapes; vinaigrette made with olive oil, fresh squeezed lemon juice, apple cider vinegar (Giant), ground mustard seed, black pepper and salt

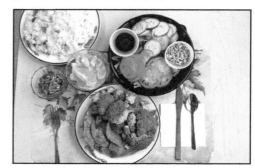

Dinner: Beef tender roast (Tyson); rice pilaf (Roland), garlic, onions, sweet peppers and olive oil); steamed broccoli; salad (green leaf lettuce, tomatoes, cucumbers) with balsamic vinaigrette (Nature's Promise); orange slices; pecans, salt & pepper

To ensure that the processed diet wasn't just obvious junk foods, Hall's team served highly processed foods that a "typical" American might eat daily and possibly consider nutritious, like Cheerios, blueberry muffins and orange juice for breakfast; cheese and turkey sandwiches with baked Lay's potato chips and diet lemonade for lunch; and steak, canned corn, mashed potatoes from a packet, and a diet beverage at dinner.

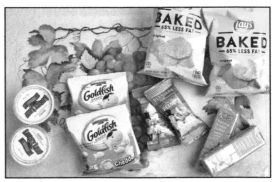

Subjects on the processed diet were also offered snacks like low-fat chips, Pepperidge Farm Goldfish crackers and other packaged foods typically found in vending machines.
Photographs: Paule Joseph and Shavonne Pocock

Results

The most striking finding was that the *ultra-processed* diet led subjects to consume 508 extra calories a day, resulting in an average of two pounds of weight gain (*a pound of that was pure fat*) in just two weeks! On the flip side, when the subjects were on the unprocessed diet, they ended up losing about two pounds over two weeks.

On the *unprocessed* diet, the subjects got their fibre, sugar and carbs from fresh produce, beans, oatmeal, sweet potatoes, grains and other whole foods.

On the *ultra-processed* diet, they ate mainly refined carbs and added sugars found in bread, bagels, juices, tater tots, sauces, chips, pasta, French fries and canned foods. The subjects were given fibre supplements on the processed diet because those foods are typically low in fibre.

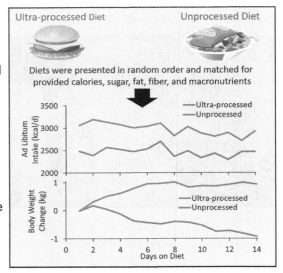

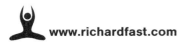

In addition to the weight gained on the ultra-processed food diet, subject's body-fat mass increased by almost 1 pound.

An analysis of their hormone levels seemed to indicate why: On the **unprocessed** diet, they had higher levels of an appetite-suppressing hormone called PPY, which is secreted by the gut, and lower levels of ghrelin, a hunger hormone, which might explain why they ate fewer calories.

On the **ultra-processed** diet, these hormonal changes flipped. Hence, participants had lower levels of the appetite-suppressing hormone and higher levels of the hunger hormone. (13)

Observations

Study participants were allowed to eat as much or as little as they wanted but ended up eating way more of the ultra-processed meals, even though they didn't rate those meals as tastier than the unprocessed meals, which eliminated taste as a factor for greater consumption.

Another interesting finding: Both groups ate about the same amount of protein, but those on the ultra-processed diet ate a lot more carbs and fat.

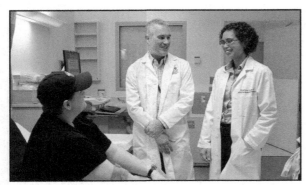

Researchers from the National Institutes of Health: Kevin D. Hall, Ph.D., center, and Stephanie Chung, M.B.B.S., right, talk with a study participant at the NIH Clinical Center.
Photo: Jennifer Rymaruk, NIDDK

There is a concept called the *protein leverage hypothesis* that suggests that people will eat until they've met their protein needs.

Hall says that this seems to be the case in this study, and it partially explains the difference in calorie consumption. (18)

Even though the meals were matched for calories and nutrients, including protein,

OBESITY *It's NOT what YOU THINK it is!*

the ultra-processed meals were more calorie-dense per bite. In part, that's because ultra-processed foods tend to be low in fibre, so researchers had to add fibre to the beverages served as part of these meals to match the fibre content of the unprocessed diet. That means participants on the ultra-processed diet might have had to munch through more carbs and fat to hit their protein needs.

And one last finding of note: People ate much faster — both in terms of grams per minute and calories per minute — on the ultra-processed diet. Hall says it might be that, because the ultra-processed foods tended to be softer and easier to chew, people devoured them more quickly, so they didn't give their gastrointestinal tracts enough time to signal to their brains that they were full and ended up overeating.

"The difference in weight gain for one [group] and weight loss for the other during these two periods is phenomenal. We haven't seen anything like this. The take-home message for consumers is we should try to eat as much real food as we can. That can be plant food. It can be animal food. It can be [unprocessed] beef, pork, chicken, fish or vegetables and fruits. And one has to be very careful once one begins to go into other kinds of food." (18)

Barry Popkin, Nutrition Professor, University of North Carolina

"These are landmark findings that the processing of the foods makes a huge difference in how much a person eats. What was so impressive was that the NIH researchers documented this weight gain even though each meal offered on the two different diets contained the same amount of calories, fats, protein, sugar, salt, carbohydrates and fibre. That's important because the majority of foods now sold in the U.S. — and increasingly, around the globe — are ultra-processed." (18)

Dariush Mozaffarian, Dean of Tufts University's Friedman School of Nutrition Science

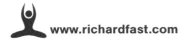

3 "Scientific" Studies Confirm
Ultra-Processed Food Drives Obesity

Study #2

How to Lose 12-Pounds of FAT,
Without Counting a Single Calorie!

One of the more meaningful weight-loss studies I've come across was reported in 2018 in *The Journal of American Medicine*, which published the results of a randomized clinical trial on the difference between a low-fat diet and a low-carb diet, and it went by the "riveting" title of;

"Effect of Low-Fat vs Low-Carbohydrate Diet on 12-Month Weight Loss in Overweight Adults and the Association With Genotype Pattern or Insulin Secretion" ... okay then.

On the surface, this study looked like so many others. Still, the excitement of the title notwithstanding, not only were the results surprising, but the researchers got an entirely different outcome than they had anticipated.

The study was led by Christopher Gardner, the director of nutrition studies at the *Stanford Prevention Research Center.*

Dr. Gardner and his colleagues designed the study to compare how overweight and obese people fare on low-carbohydrate and low-fat diets. In addition, researchers wanted to test the hypothesis that some people are predisposed to do better on one diet over the other, depending on their genetics and their ability to metabolize carbs and fat. (19)

The Study

This study involved 609 participants whose median age was 40; all were overweight but were free of all primary health concerns, in other words, no diabetes, cancer, heart disease, high cholesterol and so on.

The most striking thing about this clinical trial were the two major concepts:

> 1. All 609 participants were told there were no calorie restrictions so they could eat as much as they wanted, whether assigned to the low-carb diet or the low-fat diet, and

> 2. A dietitian regularly counseled all participants to eat whole foods rather than processed foods for a full 12 months.

In other words, it didn't matter if they were on the low-fat diet or the low-carb diet; the key was to eat whole foods that were minimally processed, nutrient-dense, and cooked at home whenever possible. (20)

Critical Points for the Low-Fat Dieters

For example, soft drinks, fruit juice, muffins, white rice, and white bread are technically low in fat. Still, the low-fat diet group was told to avoid those things and eat foods like brown rice, barley, steel-cut oats, lentils, lean meats, low-fat dairy products, quinoa, fresh fruit and legumes.

Critical Points for the Low-Carb Dieters

The low-carb group was trained to choose nutritious foods like olive oil, salmon, avocados, hard cheeses, vegetables, nut butter, nuts and seeds, and grass-fed and pasture-raised animal foods.

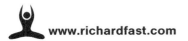

The Results

At the end of 12 months, the results were nothing short of astonishing.

Four hundred and eighty-one participants completed the trial. Some people gained weight, and some lost 50 to 60 pounds, but the average weight loss was 12 pounds. Not only that, but they saw improvements in their waist size, body fat composition, blood sugar and blood pressure levels.

The researchers admitted they were somewhat surprised at the findings because their purpose had been to study the effects of a high-quality, low-fat diet versus a high-quality low-carb diet, but as the results clearly showed, the type of diet was irrelevant. The only critical factor was that the participants ate real food.

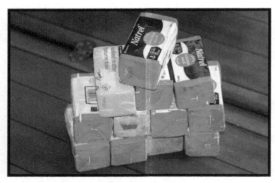

The density of butter is just a tiny bit denser than body fat. So, if you're wondering what 12 pounds of fat actually looks like, wonder no more!

Consider that for a moment; the participants could eat as much food as they wanted for an entire year and yet they still lost an average of 12 pounds ... and that's not water weight; that's 12 pounds of pure fat!

"A couple of weeks into the study, people were asking when we were going to tell them how many calories to cut back on," recalled Dr. Gardner. "Many of the people in the study were surprised — and relieved — that they did not have to restrict or even think about calories." (21)

"We explained that if what they were doing left them feeling hungry, then when they achieved their weight-loss goal, or the study ended, they would likely go off their diet and back

OBESITY... It's NOT what YOU THINK it is!

to what they were eating before, and so the weight would likely come back on." (22)

"We wanted them to find a new eating pattern they could maintain forever, without even thinking of it as a diet. We got a lot of positive feedback from the participants: they were happy not to count calories or limit their daily caloric intake."

"The most common type of feedback we got from the most successful participants (in both diet groups) was that we had 'changed their relationship to food.'" (22)

What's key was emphasizing that these were healthy low-fat and low-carb diets: A soda might be low-fat, but it's certainly not healthy. Lard may be low-carb, but an avocado would be healthier.

In addition to teaching the participants (in 22 evening classes spread out over the year of the study) about low vs. high carb and fat intakes, we also worked with all participants on mindful vs. mindless eating. For example we asked them to not eat in the car or in front of a screen, to eat with friends and family, to try to cook for them and with them more often, and to shop more frequently for ingredients at a local market ... and don't buy ultra-processed convenience food crap! (19)

Stop Counting Calories and Lose Weight?

Calorie counting has long been ingrained in the overall nutrition and weight loss advice.

"I think one place we go wrong," said Dr. Gardner, "is telling people to figure out how many calories they eat and then telling them to cut back on 500 calories, which makes them miserable. We need to focus on that foundational diet, which is more vegetables, more whole foods, less added sugar and less refined grains."

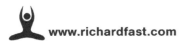 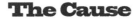

It's not that calories don't matter. After all, both groups ultimately consumed fewer calories on average by the end of the study, even though they were not conscious of it. The point is that they did this by focusing on nutritious whole foods that satisfied their hunger.

The Takeaway

"Perhaps the biggest takeaway from this study," Gardner said, "is that the fundamental strategy for losing weight with either a low-fat or low-carb approach is similar. Eat less sugar, less refined flour and as many vegetables as possible. Go for whole foods, whether that is a wheatberry salad or grass-fed beef. On both sides, we heard from people who have lost the most weight that we had helped them change their relationship to food and that now they were more thoughtful about how they ate."

Taking Control

We are being programmed to consume nutrient-void, processed junk whose only purpose is to nourish the financial health of the Big Food companies.

If we capitulate to the influence and manipulation of Big Food, if we allow them to manage our diet and trick us into excessive consumption of ultra-processed junk, we're going to pay a terrible price in terms of our health and well-being.

So, here's the thing; how much would your life change if you manage your diet with this simple declaration; *from now on, I'm only eating real food!*

Declare that, and you're beginning to understand what health and weight mastery is all about.

3 "Scientific" Studies Confirm
Ultra-Processed Food Drives Obesity

Study #3

What Are We Feeding Our Kids?
Eating Junk Food for One Month
Took Ten Years Off My Life!

Chris van Tulleken, an infectious diseases doctor for the *University College London Hospital* subjected himself to a gruelling self-experiment; for 28 days, he ate a strict diet of frozen pizza, fried chicken, fish sticks, cereals, and other ready-made meals. (23)

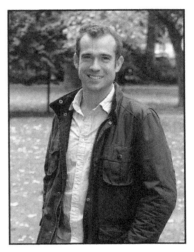

As Dr. van Tulleken said, "It sounds extreme, but it's the diet of one in five people in the UK, and I wanted to find out what effect a diet high in ultra-processed food would have on me." (24)

His results were chronicled in a 2021 BBC documentary titled, "What Are We Feeding Our Kids? (25)

It's Not a Lack of Moral Fibre,
It About What's Available to Eat

The documentary begins with van Tulleken at the *Queen Alexandra Hospital* in Portsmouth. We see Dr. Shaw Somers performing weight-loss surgery on a patient who's been overweight most of his childhood and is now 23. The surgery involves removing a large portion of his stomach.

Following the surgery, van Tulleken asks Dr. Somers how he feels about the obesity problem that's been slowly creeping up for a long time.

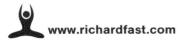

With a surprised look on his face, Somers replies,

"I wouldn't so much say slowly creeping up. It's been heading to us like an express train. Pretty soon, it's going to hit home what we're going to have; instead of just very overweight adults, we're going to have a whole cohort of very overweight children looking forward to a lifetime of ill health. And that alone should ring alarm bells."

Dr van Tulleken then asks Somers if this is a case of personal responsibility.

"It's a minor part of the whole problem," says Somers. "I think personal responsibility is not the way to tackle the obesity pandemic. Human nature really hasn't changed; what's changed is our food environment. The kind of foods that you can buy, the way they're prepared, that's what's changed. People haven't suddenly lost moral fibre over the last 20 or 30 years. Ask anyone who's tried dieting – they really try. It's about what is there available for you to eat?"

Collecting "BEFORE" Experiment Data

The purpose of the month-long experiment was to see if changing his diet from 20 percent ultra-processed foods to 80 percent ultra-processed foods would affect his health.

To ensure the results were scientifically valid, he enlisted the help of Dr. Rachel Batterham, a professor of obesity, diabetes, and endocrinology at *University College London*.

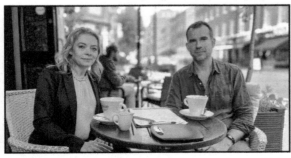

Dr Rachel Batterham and Dr Chris van Tulleken Source: BBC

To get a detailed picture of Chris's health initially, Dr. Batterham recorded his weight, fat percentage, and the levels of his hunger and satiety hormones. In addition, he was given an MRI scan to map the connections in his brain to see if eating more ultra-processed foods would change his brain activity and appetite control because if ultra-processed food is addictive, then it should act on the same parts of the brain as alcohol, drugs and cigarettes.

Chris van Tulleken Begins His Month-long Experiment

Beginning Day One with a breakfast of fried chicken, he spent the next 28 days stuffing his face with "hyper-palatable" food items. Although he loved the taste of the food, it wasn't long before his body started to suffer.

Within days, he noticed changes. Firstly, he ate much more than he was used to.

"When I was eating unprocessed food, I usually ate three meals a day with the occasional snack," he said. "With ultra-processed food, I found myself eating all the time; it simply wasn't enough.

The stuffed-crust pizza I had in the second week wasn't that delicious, but I just couldn't put it down."

Overall, he just felt really unwell. Not surprisingly, he was constipated since ultra-processed food is typically low in fibre, which caused him to develop piles. Then in the third week, he experienced sleep problems. The piles itched and kept him awake. The high salt intake was also waking him up, which caused a need to pee or to get something to drink. In addition to all that, he started suffering from heartburn, high anxiety, and his libido was virtually non-existent. (26)

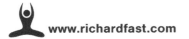

The Results

By Day 29, Chris' weight had increased by nearly 15 pounds, and his body fat alone increased by 6.6 pounds. The rest was made up of carbs stored in his liver and

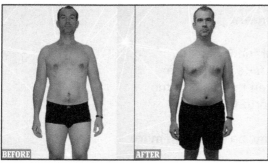

Source: BBC

muscles. His body mass index (BMI) jumped by two points which took him from normal into the overweight range.

Chris surmised, "If I'd carried on this way for a year, my weight could have almost doubled. But what was most surprising was what happened to my appetite hormones, with a 30 percent increase in hunger hormones and a similarly significant decrease in the hormones that should make me feel full and stop eating."

However, the most striking and alarming changes were seen in his brain by comparing brain scans conducted before and after the experiment.

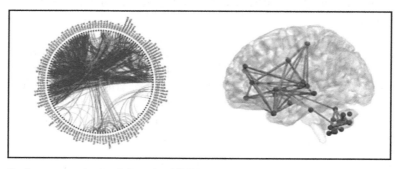

Brain scans showed that the UPF diet had created new links in his brain from areas responsible for reward to areas that drive automatic and repetitive behaviour. *Source: BBC*

Dr. Batterham: *"Blue is how areas of your brain talked to each other before the diet. And the red are the new functional brain connections in your brain after four weeks on the diet. So everything that's red is a new connection between parts of your brain that wasn't there before."*

OBESITY It's NOT what YOU THINK it is!

"The diet has linked up the reward centres of my brain with the areas that drive repetitive, automatic behaviour," explains van Tulleken. "So eating ultra-processed food has become something my brain simply tells me to do without me even wanting it. This is something you might see in a person with an addiction." *

After the Experiment

To Chris, the results were so shocking, he's stopped eating ultra-processed foods altogether.

"At home, we now ensure that our children – our baby and the four-year-old – just eat normal food, rather than highly processed baby foods and children's meals."

Chris finished his experiment in October 2020, and since then (6 months later), he has gradually lost all of his gained weight. As he said, "I have a big appetite, so it's a steady but slow process. Mercifully, my piles got better within weeks, and my heartburn and anxiety stopped almost overnight. I knew I had to go cold turkey on ultra-processed foods because, as I learned during the experiment, they are like an addictive substance: if your brain gets wired to addictiveness for it, you can't moderate your intake; you'll just crave more. That same story will already be a lifelong one for countless British children, teens and young people."

*8 weeks after starting the experiment and 4 weeks after it was over, Dr. van Tulleken had a third MRI scan. This showed that the changes in his brain were still apparent; the situation did not return to its pre-experiment state.

"I have 2 small children, and I worry a lot", he said, "if this food can change my brain in 4 weeks, what is it doing to the developing brain of my 4-year-old?"

~ Chris van Tulleken

A Candid Interview with the
Food and Drink Federation

Near the end of the documentary, Dr van Tulleken says he's keen to share his results with the food industry itself, so he met with Tim Rycroft, the chief operating officer of the *Food and Drink Federation*. They represent some of the biggest manufacturers. (25)

Dr Chris van Tulleken

What is the role and responsibility that the food industry has in the obesity epidemic and particularly with regard to children? Do you accept any responsibility for it?

Tim Rycroft

Yes, of course. Diet is one of the factors that drive obesity, and of course, the food that we eat, the pattern of food we eat over time, and the exercise that we get, are major factors contributing to overweight and obesity. I think we're doing a lot, I don't think it's enough. Clearly, it's not enough because the burden of obesity is still very high and stubbornly high. So absolutely we accept responsibility, and we have to do more. But I don't think foods are intrinsically harmful. I think bad diets are intrinsically harmful and we need to help people make those choices.

Dr Chris van Tulleken

But I put it to you that the main driver of choice about food is the food that's available, the price of that food, and then the marketing of that food. All of which are, of course, your area of expertise. So if you're faced with a choice, a true choice, between profit and public health, what's the priority?

Tim Rycroft

Well the priority's profit. The question is, can you bring those two interests together? We need to work hard to ensure that consumers are able to make great choices and that they're supported and educated about the consequences of the choices they're making because clearly, people are not making the right diet choices at the moment, when you look at the obesity figures.

OBESITY *It's NOT what YOU THINK it is!*

Dr Chris van Tulleken	*What do you think of ultra-processed foods?*
Tim Rycroft	*Well, it's not a definition I accept. There isn't a scientifically agreed definition, as opposed to something like high fat, salt, sugar, which has a clear definition.*
Dr Chris van Tulleken	*It's quite widely recognized scientifically. There are several countries that have it in their national guidelines; it's recognized by the World Health Organization.*
Tim Rycroft	*There is no internationally agreed definition.*
Dr Chris van Tulleken	*Well, I would say there is. I'm just surprised you say it's just not scientifically agreed, wherein the peer-reviewed literature, there is an agreed definition, recognized by people like Cancer Research UK.*
Tim Rycroft	*Well, it's accepted by all the critics of the food industry.* (25)

The Takeaway

We began this *Part III* by acknowledging that *"one's"* obesity can result from many things; economics, social science, psychology, biology, nutrition, endocrinology, willpower, habit and just about anything else we want to throw in the mix.

However, we also recognized that there had to be an identifiable cause for entire populations to suddenly become overweight. That meant we had to answer several questions such as:

> *The human animal is adapted to, and apparently can thrive on, an extraordinary range of different diets, but the Western diet, however you define it, does not seem to be one of them.*
>
> ~ Michael Pollan

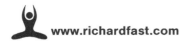

- How is it that people who were overweight stood out from the general population for thousands of years?
- Why did obesity suddenly begin in the mid-70s in the USA and indiscriminately affect millions of people? (1)
- Although the speed and extent of weight gain varied somewhat by age, gender, and ethnicity, why did all subgroups become heavier at the same time? (2)
- While, on average, all Americans were getting heavier since the mid-80s, why were the heaviest people gaining disproportionately more weight than the others?

The overwhelming *scientific* evidence in answer to the above is *ultra-processed food*.

Is Obesity Caused by Design?

It's safe to say that Big Food Companies don't deliberately design ultra-processed food to make us obese. Obesity results from their design of ultra-processed food. Their intent is profit. The result is our global obesity pandemic.

In the next part, (*The Cure*) we'll look at what we can do to slow, stop and even reverse the debilitating effects of obesity.

References

1. Reither, E.N., Hauser, R.M., Yang, Y., "Do Birth Cohorts Matter? Age-Period-Cohort Analyses of the Obesity Epidemic in the United States," Soc Sci Med 2009; 69:1439-1448
2. Rodgers, A., Woodward, A., Swinburn, B., Dietz, W. H., "Prevalence Trends Tell Us What Did Not Precipitate the US Obesity Epidemic," The Lancet, Vol. 3, April 2018
3. Young, L. R., Nestle, M., "Expanding Portion Sizes in the US Marketplace: Implications for Nutrition Counseling," J Am. Diet Assoc., 2003;103:231-240
4. Bleich, S. N., Cutler, D., Murray, C., Adams, A., "Why is the Developed World Obese?" Annu. Rev Public Health, 2008; 29:273-295
5. Huber, B., "Welcome to Brazil Where a Food Revolution is Changing the Way People Eat: How the Country Challenged the Junk-Food Industry and Became a Global Leader in the Battle Against Obesity," The Nation, July 28, 2016

6. Dietary Guidelines for the Brazilian Population, 2nd Edition 2014

7. Rear, J., "How to Identify 'Ultra-Processed Foods – The Grub That's Linked to Death," The Telegraph, May 30, 2019

8. Monteiro, C., et al. "Ultra-Processed Foods: What They Are and How to Identify Them," Cambridge University Press, Feb. 12, 2019

9. Duke Sanford, World Food Policy Center, Podcast E24: Carlos Monteiro on the Dangers of Ultra-Processed Foods

10. Monteiro, C., et al., "The UN Decade of Nutrition, the NOVA Food Classification and the Trouble with Ultra-Processing," Public Health Nutr. 2018 Jan;21(1):5-17

11. Tufts University, "Ultra-processed Foods Now Comprise 2/3 of Calories in Children and Teen Diets, Science Daily, August 10, 2021

12. Crowe, K., "Food Cravings Engineered by Industry: How Big Food Keeps Us Eating Through a Combination of Science and Marketing," CBC News, March 6, 2013

13. Moss, M., "Salt Sugar Fat: How the food Giants Hooked Us," Random House Canada, Toronto, 2013

14. Moss, M., "Hooked: Food, Free Will, and How the Food Giants Exploit Our Addictions," Random House Canada, Toronto, 2021

15. Kluger, J., "Food Addictions Are Real Addictions – and More and More People Are Getting Hooked," TIME: The Science of Addiction – What We Know. What We're Learning, Nov 6, 2019

16. Gearhardt, A, Hebebrand, J., "The Concept of "Food Addiction" Helps Inform the Understanding of Overeating and Obesity: YES," Am. J Clin Nutr., 2021 Feb 2; 113(2):263-267

17. Schulte, E., Avena, N. M., Gearhardt, A. N., "Which Foods May Be Addictive? The Roles of Processing, Fat Content, and Glycemic Load," PLoS One, 2015;10(2): e0117959

18. Hall K., et al., "Ultra-Processed Diets Cause Excess Calorie Intake and Weight Gain: An Inpatient Randomized Controlled Trial of Ad Libitum Food Intake," Cell Metabolism, July 2, 2019, Vol. 30:67-77

19. Armitage, H., "Low-Fat or Low-Carb? It's a Draw, Study Finds," Stanford Medicine, News, Feb. 20, 2018

20. Gardner, C. D., et al., "Effect of Low-Fat vs Low-Carbohydrate Diet on 12-Month Weight Loss in Overweight Adults and the Association with Genotype Pattern or Insulin Secretion," JAMA, 2018 Feb 20; 319(7):667-679

21. O'Connor, A., "The Key to Weight Loss is Diet Quality, Not Quantity, a New Study Finds," New York Times, Feb. 20, 2018

22. Hull, M., "Low-Fat vs. Low-Carb? Major Study Concludes: It Doesn't Matter for Weight Loss," Examine.com Feb 7, 2020

23. Sparks, H., "Eating Junk Food for a Month Took 10 Years Off My Life: Doctor," New York Post, May 18, 2021

24. Chalil, M., "Cling on to Traditional Food Culture to Address Fattest Nation Reputation, UK Expert Advises Malaysians," Yahoo!News, Aug 5, 2021

25. UCL Academic Follows Ultra-Processed Food Diet for BBC Documentary, BBC, May 27, 2021

26. Mangan, L., "What Are We Feeding Our Kids? – Junk Food Exposé Will Leave You Queasy," The Guardian, May 27, 2021

27. Mercola, J., "Ultra-Processed Foods Linked to Obesity, Diabetes, Heart Disease and Cancer," The Defender, Aug 10, 2021

28. Van Tulleken, C., "Look What a Month of Eating Processed Food Did to Me! It's What Millions of US – Including Children – Eat Every Day. But as Dr Chris van Tulleken Discovered in a BBC Experiment, It's Making Us Fatter, Unhealthier ... and Even Changing Our Brains," The Daily Mail, May 17, 2021

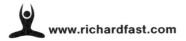

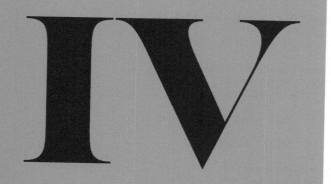

part IV

The Cure

Cure ~ *To restore to health,*
soundness, or normality.
Merriam-Webster

Your health is your only tether to life on this planet. When your health is gone, you're gone. That pretty much makes it your most valuable possession, and yet, many people fail to make regular investments in their health.

Part of the reason may be that we take our health for granted, but I believe a more significant reason is a lack of understanding of what health is and how to achieve it.

Ultra-processed food is the primary cause of our obesity pandemic, but the cure will require more than a fixation on ultra-processed foods alone. To overcome the formidable forces of obesity, we need to think in terms of our total health, which requires three things:

➤ A better understanding of what it means to be healthy

➤ Adjust our thinking about diet and obesity, because a simple change in perspective can transform our habits, behaviours, beliefs, and results

➤ Develop a better appreciation for food ... real food

First, let's look at what it means to be healthy.

The Cure for Obesity is Not to Focus on Weight; It's to Focus on Health

I'll begin with a question: Do you like your body? I'm serious, do you *really* like it? Oh sure, we'd all love to have bodies like the models gracing the covers of fitness magazines, but wishful thinking aside, how much do you care about looking after the body you have?

When people decide to lose weight and are asked their goal, they often cite a weight-loss plan up to three times greater than what a doctor might recommend. Given how difficult that can be to pull off, it's no wonder that so many people give up trying to lose weight altogether. But most people do not need to lose quite so much to improve their health. Research shows that with just a 10% loss of weight (fat), people will experience noticeable changes in their blood pressure and blood sugar control, while lowering their risk for heart disease and Type 2 diabetes – two of the costliest diseases in terms of health and quality of life. [1]

There's No Such Thing As a Healthy Weight, Only a Healthy Person

As a society, we've been conditioned to think that being "thin" is a sure sign of health, while being "overweight" (according to the BMI charts) signals significant health issues. Is this true?

Not necessarily, because the fact is, you can be so-called overweight and still be far healthier than many so-called thin people.

➤ So, what are the health implications of being fit or unfit?

➤ What does it mean to our health to be classified by the BMI (Body, Mass, Index) charts as "over-weight," "normal-weight," or "under-weight?

➤ Can we be "fit," "healthy," and "overweight" all at the same time?

The short answer to the last question is "yes," so if you've ever struggled with trying to lose weight to improve your

OBESITY,,, *It's NOT what YOU THINK it is!*

health, this part is going to be a wellspring of good news! Now don't get me wrong, losing fat and improving body composition is a beautiful goal. Still, it's your level of *fitness*, not *fatness*, that plays the most significant role in ensuring your health and vitality.

I don't believe that any book discussing obesity, and its cure, should ignore the critical importance of exercise to our overall health.

Exercise is the single best thing you can do for yourself. It's way more important than dieting and easier to do. Exercise works at so many levels — except one: your weight.

~ Robert Lustig, Fat Chance: Beating the Odds Against Sugar, Processed Food, Obesity and Disease

We've Been Led to Believe (Wrongly) that Being "Overweight" is a Direct Cause of Premature Death

Many studies have "set out" to determine the role of so-called "overweight" in illness and premature death, however, it may come as a surprise that even though "overweight" is frequently sighted as a significant cause of mortality, being "overweight" does not *necessarily* contribute to premature death. In other words, association does not automatically equate to causation. While it's true that many overweight people suffer from poor health and premature death, so do many people who are considered normal or underweight. (2)

To illustrate the folly of equating *association* with *causation*, researcher John Yudkin published a tongue-in-cheek study in 1957 showing that television and radio ownership was a far more significant cause of coronary mortality in England than any dietary factor. In other words, he facetiously claimed that the principal cause of heart disease was mere ownership of a radio or television because the correlation between the two was statistically overwhelming! (3)

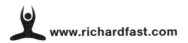 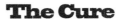

Radios and televisions cannot cause heart disease, but they could lead to a drastic reduction in physical activity compared to those who didn't own a radio or television.

One of the first studies on the relationship between physical activity and mortality rates was done in 1864 in London, England. The study compared the health of sedentary tailors with the active lifestyle of agricultural laborers and found that mortality among tailors was much higher because of physical inactivity. (4)

Although that early study may have been scientifically inconclusive, an epidemiological study was conducted by Dr. Jeremy Morris in London, England, in 1953. Morris did several studies on various occupations and how their level of physical activity affected coronary heart disease.

Morris' most famous study was between the drivers and conductors of London's famous double-decker buses.

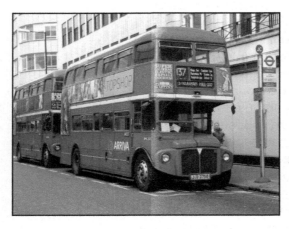

This study was so ideal because it involved several thousand subjects under identical conditions with only one variable ... physical activity.

On a London double-decker, there are only two employment positions: drivers and conductors. The actual shift was 5 ½ hours long, during which drivers, on average, sat for 90% of their shift, and conductors sat for less than 10%. Conservatively, the conductors climbed 500-750 stairs per working day, which has been compared to brief interval training. Mean heart rate during a working shift was 106 beats per minute in conductors and 91 beats per minute in drivers. (5)

Although the study was focused on the effects of physical

OBESITY *It's NOT what YOU THINK it is!*

activity on coronary heart disease, Morris and his colleagues also wanted to know if body size played a role in the results. Surprisingly ... or not, it didn't!

All the drivers and conductors wore uniforms, so their pants and waist size were documented. When Morris compared the pant and waist size with their cardiac mortality rates, he found no difference. The active conductors had half the cardiovascular mortality rates of sedentary drivers, regardless of whether their physique was slim, average or portly.

In addition, Dr. Morris found that the active conductors were also more than 50% less likely to die of other illnesses such as diabetes, stroke and some forms of cancer, not to mention their improved quality of life and their ability to slow the effects of aging dramatically.

Dr. Morris's double-decker study and the assertion that physical activity had a direct effect on coronary heart disease was widely met with derision, especially by the medical community!

So Dr. Morris did a follow-up study using England's postal employees. Like his previous study, this too was the gold standard of studies because it involved a wide range of people living and working in almost identical conditions with only one variable ... physical activity.

For this study, Morris compared the letter carriers to the office clerks and telephone operators. Once again, the finding clearly showed that the active carriers - regardless of their physical size or BMI - experienced half the risk of coronary heart disease as the inactive workers experienced.

Incredibly enough, despite these findings, the medical community remained highly skeptical about the links between physical activity and health, choosing instead to focus on factors such as weight-for-height ratios and lipoprotein profiles. At the same time, they completely

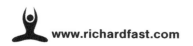

ignored Morris's findings on physical activity. In fact, the skepticism and outright criticism of Morris's findings continued in Great Britain well in the 1980s. (6)

Even today, the critical importance of regular physical activity for health takes a back-burner status in much of the medical information. A group of researchers conducted a review of medical journals read by Australian physicians between 1987 and 1997. They found that only 6% of the articles written were about physical activity, while the majority had to do with a wide variety of medications.

When reviewing the ads in these publications they were all pharmaceutical ads. (7) (Big surprise there!)

Could You Be Obese* and Not Even Know it?

Obesity is defined as: The accumulation of excessive FAT that may interfere with the maintenance of an optimal state of health.

(NOTE: it does NOT say excessive weight, it says excessive FAT)

That's why associating obesity with a BMI (Body Mass Index) of 30 or more is grossly misleading, because someone can have a BMI over 30 and still be perfectly healthy.

Many people are! In fact, 40 percent of people considered "normal" weight are actually obese! (8,9)

We tend to think that fat is fat, but that's just not so. There's "good" fat and "bad" fat, and a basic understanding of these two fats – and the cure for the bad kind – can be critical to our long-term health.

We all have fat; in fact, it's essential to life. Lean adults may have around 40 billion fat cells; in comparison, "so-called" overweight adults may have 80 to 120 billion fat cells, but here's the thing – it's not the "amount" of fat that makes the difference between being healthy and unhealthy; it's the **type of fat** and where it's distributed. (10, 11)

The "good" type of fat – known as subcutaneous fat – is found just beneath the skin, while the "bad" fat – visceral fat – is located around abdominal organs.

OBESITY... *It's NOT what YOU THINK it is!*

Subcutaneous fats have a high level of the enzyme *lipoprotein lipase*, which causes them to easily store fat and hold on to it more tightly. This means that the fat stays in the fat cells, where it is believed to positively affect health.

Visceral fat lies deep inside your abdomen and is more metabolically active than subcutaneous fat in terms of storing and releasing fat. When released into the bloodstream, it can infiltrate the liver and streak through your muscles to clog arteries and strangle your heart. Visceral fat can contribute to diabetes, heart disease, high blood pressure, strokes, and some cancers. (12,13, 14)

Are You a TOFI Person?

Professor Jimmy Bell, head of the molecular imaging group at the Medical Research Council's Centre at Imperial College, has spent years studying how human beings store and use their adipose tissue (fat). He has carried out studies showing that people considered slim can have large quantities of fat within them. As Bell noted;

> *We've scanned underweight people and found up to seven litres of fat inside them. Someone who appears thin on the outside yet doesn't exercise may be at risk of a host of health problems because their fat is stored on the inside and in the organs. This is particularly true for men who have a slim build but do little or no exercise. We know now that 40 percent of people have fat infiltration of the liver, which is linked to so many other health problems. (8)*

Thanks to the latest MRI (magnetic resonance imaging) techniques, we can understand why appearances can be so deceiving and why so many people can be described as a 'TOFI' – ***Thin on the Outside, Fat on the Inside***.

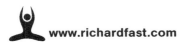 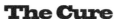

Similar Age, Gender, BMI and Same % Body Fat

Different levels of Internal Fat = Different Disease Risks

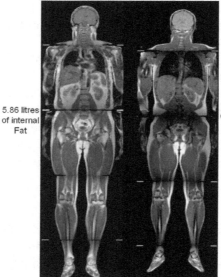

5.86 litres of internal Fat

1.65 litres of internal fat

EL Thomas and JD Bell 2008

The figure illustrates two men, both 35 years old, with a BMI of 25 kg/m2. Despite their similar size, the TOFI had 5.86 litres of internal fat, whilst the healthy control had only 1.65 litres. (8)

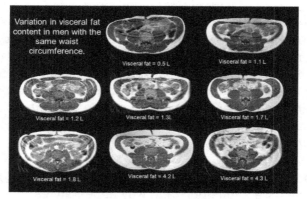

Variation in visceral fat in men with the same waist circumference

To classify an individual as TOFI, it is essential to measure their internal fat content. MRI or CT scanning, show fat as bright (white) and lean tissue as dark. The figure clearly shows that despite having an identical waist circumference (in this example all men had a waist of 84 cm), there is considerable variation in the amount of visceral fat (volumes shown on the image in litres) present. (8)

OBESITY... It's NOT what YOU THINK it is!

Although the only way to know for sure if fat is encapsulating your vital organs is to get lab tests and MRI scans, a quick way to guesstimate if you are TOFI is to measure your waist to hip ratio (WHR). Ideally, you want your waist to be smaller than your hips. Signs of abdominal obesity; your WHR is greater than or equal to 0.9 for a man and greater than or equal to 0.85 for a woman.

When It Comes to Fat, Don't Always Believe What You See!

Both the public and the medical community often get sidetracked by BMI, a method of measuring fat developed 150 years ago in Belgium. BMI is calculated under the metric system by taking your weight in kilograms and dividing it by your height in metres squared.

The problem with BMI is that it really doesn't work individually. For example, studies have found that, for the most part, professional athletes such as a 350-pound football player or a 500-pound Sumo wrestler are metabolically healthy because they have surprisingly low levels of visceral fat.

Sumo wrestlers have been put through MRI scanners, and even though they have a BMI of 56 and are eating up to 5,000 calories a day, they have very little internal fat. These people are "fit," which means they generally have low cholesterol, low triglycerides, and low insulin resistance. Their fat is predominantly subcutaneous – the fat stored under the skin on the outside.

Your body shape "can" be a telltale sign about the type of fat your body stores. If you have an "apple" shaped body – fat around your belly rather than below your waist – you're more likely to have a higher level of visceral body fat. If, instead, you have a "pear" shaped body – your fat tends to gather on your thighs and hips – you're more likely to get benefits from your fat. (15, 16, 17, 18, 19, 20)

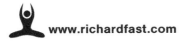

Be Skeptical When Reading Media Headlines

Unfortunately, a number of epidemiological studies on health and fitness have been misinterpreted by the media. They tend to make broad – and erroneous – conclusions about fat and its effect on our health without making the critical distinction between types of fat. Even worse, some studies were based on the sketchy measuring stick of BMI. From that basis, we could easily conclude that "overweight" people were unfit and unhealthy. In contrast, thin people were generally fit and healthy.

New studies unequivocally conclude that it's not "fat" in general that poses the most significant health risks, but rather the type of fat and where it's located.

The first way to manipulate the way your body stores fat is diet; reduce the consumption of ultra-processed foods to as close to zero as possible. The second way is to get sufficient exercise.

But then again, I suspect you already knew that.

All We Need is a Good Pair of Walking Shoes!

Not surprisingly, the bottom line is - and it's always about the bottom line; there's no money to be made if all we need is a good pair of walking shoes!

A 1989 study was published that analyzed the records of more than 10,000 men and 3,000 women who had taken a treadmill fitness test. Each of these testers was then monitored for the following eight years.

The findings were indisputable; low physical fitness was a health risk factor for men and women. High levels of physical activity appeared to delay all-cause mortality. The study concluded that heavier individuals who were fit and fat had far lower death rates than thin but unfit people. (21)

In 1999, Dr. Wei and his colleagues published the most extensive study ever done on the effects of physical activity and mortality rates. The study involved over 25,000 participants who had received a complete physical examination and a treadmill fitness test between 1970 and 1993, with a mortality follow-up to December 31, 1994.

The following graphics show all-cause mortality rates for each BMI group broken down by levels of fitness and BMI. According to the "accepted" definitions of BMI, average weight is 18.5 to 24.9% body fat; overweight is 25.0 to 29.9% body fat, and obese is classed as 30.0% or higher.

Fitness vs. Fatness in All-Cause Mortality

Mortality Rate

	Fit	Sedentary
BMI under 25	1	2.2
BMI 25 - 30	1.1	2.5
BMI over 30	1.1	3.1

Let's take a moment and review this chart. The one thing you can't help but notice is that "fitness" reduced all-cause mortality by approximately 50% regardless of BMI! (22)

If you want to increase your health span and quality of life, your first goal is to get yourself as fit as possible and let your BMI become a secondary issue.

If you have a BMI under 25 and you're unfit, you have at least twice the all-cause mortality rate as anyone who is fit, regardless of BMI. If your BMI is over 30 and you're unfit, you have about three times the all-cause mortality rate as anyone who is fit.

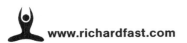

So the bottom line is pretty straightforward: Get fit, eat real food, and everything else, including your weight, will fall into place. I can't help but think that this is terrific news because studies show that you really can have your proverbial cake and eat it too; all you have to do is put your priorities in the proper order. And here's that order:

1. Health
2. Fitness
3. Body Composition

There is one immutable law of exercise; doing "something" is better than doing nothing.

By making health and fitness a priority, you will automatically focus on things over which you have complete control rather than chasing after a potentially impossible body type. Some of us were born endomorphs, naturally having a heavier, thicker body type. Others are naturally lean ectomorphs. The remainder is classed as mesomorphs, who fall somewhere in the middle.

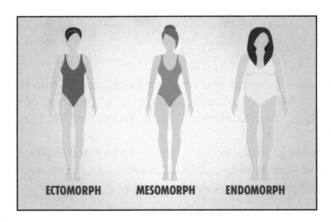

ECTOMORPH   **MESOMORPH**   **ENDOMORPH**

You cannot change your body type, but you can give your body every opportunity to remain healthy, youthful and vigorous.

OBESITY *It's NOT what YOU THINK it is!*

By focusing on what you can control, you will automatically make better dietary and fitness choices, leading to slightly better habits. These subtle changes happen so quietly that you may not even notice, but it's the slight changes in lifestyle that result in massive change over time.

Exercise affects virtually every cell, organ and system in your body. A single exercise session can turn on numerous genes in the activated muscles that affect the entire body. Your skeletal muscles produce countless "drug-like" molecules, like proteins and growth factors, resulting in beneficial systemic effects. (23, 24)

Although the "fit but fat" phenotype may be rare, it's mainly because people with a high BMI don't often participate in physical activity.

Studies continually show that the beneficial effects of exercise on aerobic capacity, glucose metabolism, blood pressure, lipids, vascular function and inflammatory markers result from physical activity regardless of one's BMI. (25, 26)

I hope you can embrace the indisputable fact that <u>thin</u> isn't fit; FIT IS FIT!

To Reverse Global Obesity, We Must Change Our Perspective

Many years ago, I had a 60-cigarette per day addiction that lasted for almost 15 years. I tried to quit using every remedy known; I tried cutting back, cold turkey, willpower, acupuncture, and even hypnosis. I would usually manage to "quit" for a few days or weeks, but I always returned.

The Circular Dilemma

While I was smoking, I hated it and wanted to quit. When I quit, all I could think about was my desperate desire for

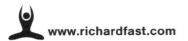

a cigarette. That's the insane contradiction of desperately wanting to quit smoking – because I knew it was killing me – while at the same time believing that life wouldn't be worth living if I quit because it would mean fighting a never-ending battle of craving and anxiety.

Perhaps you can relate. If you've battled weight loss, for example, while you're eating that seventh slice of pizza, you hate yourself for doing so. Still, when you decide to cut back on food and go on a diet, all you can think about is food, and the thought of spending the rest of your life in that agonizing state just doesn't seem worth the pain, so you say, "what the hell" and you jump off your diet with a vengeance. After several months of "overindulgence", you suddenly say, "that's it, I've had it!" and back you go to trying the latest fad diet or exercise program that promises to solve all your weight-loss problems.

That's the circular dilemma that we get caught in when we try to change a behaviour without changing our perspective. We desperately want to change our present behaviour, but when we try using willpower and teeth-gritted effort, it suddenly seems more painful than maintaining the status quo.

"You" Have to Change, BEFORE "You" Can Change

I'm going to let you in on a simple secret; as long as you try to change a habit or addiction by using gimmicks – in my case, willpower, hypnosis, acupuncture, nicotine gum and so on – you are essentially the same person, with the same thoughts, feelings, fears and beliefs, only now you're pinning your hopes on a "new" distraction; a fad diet, an exercise contraption, a mantra, willpower or New Year's resolution.

When It Comes to Change, Your Belief is All that Matters

Whenever we search for obstacles to acquiring lasting behavioural change, we will always discover that it comes down to our thoughts and beliefs ... our perspective.

But here's the exciting part, because our thoughts are so formidable, the moment we see our undesirable behaviour from a different perspective, those undesirable dominant thoughts can quickly lose their grip, for good! That's the key to breaking the back of a bad habit.

Real change comes down to changing our perspective; it's about what we associate with pleasure and what we associate with ongoing pain. I was pained by smoking, but I was even more pained whenever I tried to quit. I associated a life without cigarettes as a never-ending battle of willpower and craving. You may associate losing weight with a never-ending struggle of hunger and deprivation or exercising with pain, discomfort and inconvenience. As long as those beliefs exist, lasting change is virtually impossible.

I'll Change ... But NOT Today!

Like all smokers, I always told myself that I would quit before it was too late ... whatever that meant.

Then one day, I decided that I had had enough and would finally quit for good, but I also determined that I was definitely not going to try to stop just then. From personal experience and observation, I knew that when most people decide to change some behaviour, they jump right in at the action stage, which guarantees failure because they're not really prepared. They failed to take the time and effort to change their thinking, and from my long list of failed attempts, I was acutely aware of this problem.

So, at some "non-conscious" level, I decided I would try and see this smoking thing from a different perspective. I was going to try and understand my psychological bondage. So rather than trying to cut back or stop altogether, I actually forced myself to increase my daily intake, which was no small feat when you're sucking on sixty cigarettes a day!

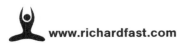

Now, this was many years ago (before *public* perspective changed), when smokers weren't looked on as the pariahs they are today. Back then (70's & 80's), you could smoke on airplanes, public transportation, (and aside from church), virtually anywhere you pleased, and nobody gave it a second thought. So, when I said I would increase my daily intake, I literally began to light one cigarette from the previous. Were there times I had just finished a cigarette and didn't feel like smoking another? Always. But I forced myself to smoke it anyway because if cigarettes are so pleasurable (I told myself), why deprive?

Overcoming The Circular Dilemma

I hated smoking while I was smoking, and when I wasn't, it was all I could think about? That was my circular dilemma. So, while I was "forcing" myself to smoke (and my nicotine levels were sky high), I could think objectively. I could think like a non-smoker because at that moment, I wasn't being driven by a desire for nicotine, and because of that, I could think clearly and rationally; in other words, I could see my habit from an objective perspective.

And so with each cigarette I smoked, I consciously thought about how much I hated my dependency. I began to look around and notice that non-smokers didn't seem to have any problem with concentration. They could effortlessly enjoy a glass of wine or cup of coffee without a cigarette. As I cleaned the snow off my car at 10:30 PM, because I was down to my last three smokes, I had to ask myself if cigarettes were the cause or cure of my anxiety.

I began to really focus on things like the smell of my clothes, my car, my breath, the yellow nicotine stains, the expense, the dirty ashtrays, and worst of all, I began to admit that this was nothing short of a very humiliating form of slavery.

At some subconscious level, I knew I was going to quit, but

I also knew that I had to let my experiment run its course ... whatever that might be.

This self-imposed torture of continually smoking more than I wanted went on for almost two weeks, and it was seriously affecting my health. I was constantly tired and felt unwell. My nicotine levels were riding sky high, and I was feeling like total crap! I had trouble breathing, I felt like throwing up, and my energy level was non-existent.

The Glorious Day Finally Arrives!

Then one morning, the most beautiful thing happened. I can recall it as clear as if it happened yesterday. I awoke and instinctively reached for my pack of cigarettes lying on the night table. As I did so, I suddenly felt that something was different. It was one of those life-defining moments because I suddenly realized I no longer had any desire to smoke.

At last, I saw my addiction for the illusion that it was, and at that moment, it no longer controlled me. I was finally free. This knowledge was so complete that I calmly picked up my cigarettes and crushed them into mush. I threw the crumpled pack in the garbage, and I haven't smoked a cigarette since. At last, I was a non-smoker, not because I didn't put a cigarette in my mouth, but because I had finally lost *all desire* to smoke.

That was thirty-five years ago.

Were there times in the ensuing weeks and months that I longed for a cigarette? Occasionally. In fact, years later, I might be talking on the phone, and the thought of "enjoying" a cigarette would pop into my mind, but the idea was fleeting and carried little substance. My freedom meant far more to me than anything else. In fact, my desire *for* a cigarette was not nearly as great as my desire to *not* have one.

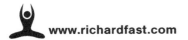

At Last, I Could Clearly See
What I was Giving Up ... Nothing!

By changing my perspective, I went from the view of giving up to getting. I wasn't going to give up smoking; I was going to start getting. I was going to start getting to enjoy my freedom; I was going to start getting to enjoy my independence, self-esteem, self-confidence, money, time, and on and on. "Giving up?" I wasn't giving up anything other than a crippling dependency. I was giving up having to go to a store late at night to buy cigarettes. I was giving up the endless smell, expense, stress, anxiety, colds, coughing fits, hacking and embarrassment.

I didn't realize it at the time, but what I had been doing during the previous two weeks – when I was forcing myself to smoke so much that my nicotine level never dropped – was teaching myself to observe my behaviour from the objective view of a non-smoker.

When my nicotine levels were sky high, I could see my habit for what it was, just like a non-smoker, and while doing so, I was laying down some powerful neuron tracks. I was challenging those deep fears that all smokers face. I was systematically dismantling the fear that quitting smoking meant living the rest of my life in constant battle.

By changing my perspective, I no longer thought about giving up; I only thought about getting. This new way of thinking was so strong, and I was so committed and adamant to free myself from my dependency, it got me through the first few days with a strong wind at my back.

What About Regression?
Why Was This Time Different?

After I threw my cigarettes away, there were inevitably a few thoughts of lighting up, but they lasted mere moments before my new thoughts would overwhelm those old

OBESITY... *It's NOT what YOU THINK it is!*

desires. The idea of having a cigarette was dealt a knockout blow before it had any chance of gaining momentum. I had finally broken the back of a bad habit.

So that's how I overcame my crippling addiction. I learned a process for overcoming my deep-seated fears and false beliefs, and this process will work for anybody in any application that requires a change in perspective. If we desire to change a behaviour but can't seem to manage, it's because we haven't changed our thoughts and beliefs about that behaviour. Our *false beliefs* bind us to behaviours we dislike or prevent us from acquiring behaviours we desire.

Why is it So Difficult to Change Our Deep-seated Habits and Beliefs?

Changing habits and beliefs isn't difficult if we follow a process of behavioural change. For example, most people fail at their weight-loss attempts because they go about it in a way that cannot succeed. They go on a calorie-restricted diet, eliminate food groups, or begin an exercise program to burn calories. Still, they fail to change the all-powerful habits and beliefs that drive their behaviour and lifestyle, so their chances of long-term success are close to zero.

Want Lasting Change? Forget About Willpower and Teeth-Gritted Effort

To this day, I will still say that my most significant accomplishment was ridding myself of the habit of smoking because I had honestly believed it was an impossibility.

However, for many years after I quit, I attributed my success to willpower and self-determination. Still, the more I thought about it, the more I realized that I had stumbled upon the real driver behind our habits and behaviours, which is our deep-seated non-conscious beliefs, and it was not until I changed my perspective that I achieved lasting results.

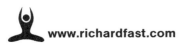

Anyone can go on a diet and lose weight. The trick is to keep the weight off for good.

If you lose weight while allowing your present thoughts and beliefs to retain their power, then it's only a matter of time until you regain the lost weight. If, however, you identify those hidden drivers that control your eating habits and you break their power, you will have acquired a permanent weapon against undesirable eating habits for the rest of your life.

Changing Our Perspective of Food

I remember back in the late '80s, and early 90's when smoking in public was just beginning to be banned. I was pretty sure the restrictions would never last because bar and restaurant owners, not to mention smokers, would never stand for it. Wow, was I wrong!

What happened? The social norm changed. It's what psychologists call a *critical perceptual shift*. Suddenly we began to see tobacco as deviant, invasive, and even repulsive. It was no longer cool to smoke. A consensus emerged that the cigarette, and the industry that manufactured it, was abhorrent. We moved from glorification to demonization. (27)

How Should We View Big Food and the Ultra-Processed Food It's Peddling?

With disdain. They manufacture wildly unhealthy products and say they're just giving us what we want. It's a mutual arrangement. But is that really true?

Did we ask them to manipulate our natural appetites? To create food that is nutrient void and addictive? Food that would virtually re-wire our brains and the brains of our children. Did we ask for food that produced ginormous profits at the expense of our health? Could we have known that a

OBESITY, *It's NOT what YOU THINK it is!*

disease – formerly known as adult-onset diabetes – would be renamed to Type II diabetes because it's now common in children? Did we ever imagine our children could be intentionally addicted to UPF and face a lifetime of obesity and ill-health?

The Big Food companies urge us to take personal responsibility for our health. Perhaps, but tell that to a 5-year-old who's being goaded into collecting all ten toys as advertised.

What happens to Your Body When You Eat Ultra-Processed Food?

What happens if you indulge in a greasy fast-food meal on occasion? Probably nothing ... other than a likely feeling of a queasy stomach and a sluggish disposition for the next couple of hours. But if ultra-processed food makes up 60 or 70 percent of your diet, be aware of what it's doing to your body — like causing weight gain, fatigue, elevated cholesterol levels, acne, depression, mood swings, bloating, addiction, increased risk for cancer – and decide whether the "convenience" of a regular diet of ultra-processed, pre-packaged food is worth the consequences.

In *The End of Overeating*, author David Kessler asked a leading food consultant to describe the ingredients in some foods commonly found in popular restaurants today.

> *Potato skins, for example: Typically, the potato is hollowed out, and the skin is fried, which provides a substantial surface area for what he calls "fat pickup." Then some combination of bacon bits, sour cream, and cheese is added. The result is fat on fat on fat on fat, much of it loaded with salt.*

> *Buffalo wings start with the fatty parts of the chicken. You load 30 to 40 percent fat when you fry it in the manufacturing plant, which pushes out 30 or 40 percent of the water. Then it's fried again in the*

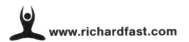

kitchen, usually of the restaurant that loads another 30 to 40 percent fat in there. Then we add the red sauce and the creamy white sauce, and what are we eating? Fat on fat on fat on fat on sugar and fat sugar and salt with a bit of protein.

"Spinach dip" is a misnomer. The spinach provides little more than colour and a bit of appeal; a high-fat, high-salt dairy product is the main ingredient. It's a tasty dish of salt on fat.

You Can Eat All Your Favorite Foods AND Enjoy a Lifetime of Health Without Counting a Single Calorie

Eating well requires a little discipline. It does NOT require willpower because you can eat as much as you like, with no restrictions when you eat natural food.

In Italy, for example, they believe in the purity of food and the wisdom of eating. They're not frightened by the joys of eating; they revere it.

Have You Ever Eaten Real Pizza?

Surprisingly enough, many Americans have no idea how pizza really tastes because they confuse it with the junk food advertised on television. In Italy, laws define pizza, which set allowances on the type of flour, tomato, mozzarella, olive oil, basil and oregano. Pizza is inherently nutritious and filling.

Street corner pizza shops in Philadelphia, New York and other large cities kept close to the original idea of simple, fresh ingredients.

Then came the pizza chains, which put most

local shops out of business. Fresh ingredients were replaced with preservative-laden, cheap and fatty ingredients that could be mass-produced, frozen and shipped across the country. Commercial pizza is now a high-calorie, high-fat, high-sodium, low-nutrient food. (15)

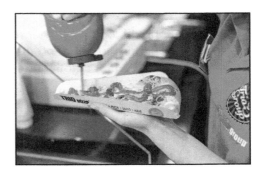

The same thing goes for milkshakes and popcorn. If you feel like a milkshake, make it with *natural* ice cream, and you'll be delightfully sated.

You don't have to avoid snacks you love. If you love salty, buttery, popcorn, make it! In fact, you may find it's as much fun to make as it is to eat! (Where have you heard that before?)

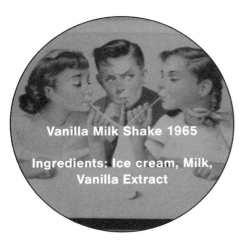

Vanilla Milk Shake 1965

Ingredients: Ice cream, Milk, Vanilla Extract

Vanilla Milk Shake 1995

Ingredients: Milk, Sugar, Cream, Corn Syrup, Natural Flavor, Mono and Diglycerides, Cellulose Gum, Guar Gum, Carrageenan, Vitamin A Palmitate, Glycerin, Caramel Color, Vanilla Extract, Natural Flavor, Salt, Potassium Sorbate (preservative), Liquid Sugar, Nitrous Oxide

If you've got a craving for pizza, avoid that frozen crap-in-a-box that's loaded with chemicals and preservatives; make a pizza using whole fresh ingredients.

Our health and weight aren't dependent on food restriction and forsaking burgers, and fries and all the other foods we love. We need to raise our standards and restore our palettes. What's more delicious than a homemade burger made with fresh whole ingredients? Or potatoes you've washed, peeled, cut into slices, drizzled with olive oil, sprinkled with spices and baked in your own oven?

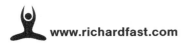

We should look down our noses at the garbage we've been conditioned to eat; food that's been so stripped of fibre and nutrients that it's nothing more than adult baby food!

"For is there any practice less selfish, any labor less alienated, any time less wasted, than preparing something delicious and nourishing for people you love?"

~ Michael Pollan

What Do You Find Acceptable?

To reverse this obesity calamity, we're going to have to change our perspective of what we consider acceptable.

When it Comes to a Healthy Diet, is It Acceptable to Let Our Children Fend for Themselves?

Although there is no shortage of doctors, nutritionists, and concerned citizens who have railed against the marketing of ultra-processed food to children and urged the government to legislate against it, the problem continues to escalate.

We can't afford to wait. Our children are becoming addicted to ultra-processed food in increasing numbers and at younger ages.

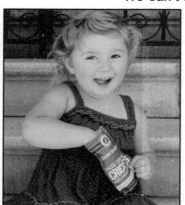

Photo: Don Bugito

As Dr. David Kessler framed it in *The End of Overeating*; *"we need to understand the implications of what is happening. If the behaviors are conditioned and driven, they can have long-term consequences."*

A two-year-old child has a natural compensation when eating. If you give a two-year-old more to eat at lunch, they'll eat less for the rest of the day ... provided they're eating real food.

OBESITY,,, *It's NOT what YOU THINK it is!*

However, by the time the "average" child is 4 or 5, they lose the ability to compensate because they're no longer eating real food, they're eating ultra-processed food, and they're eating all through the day.

Ultra-processed food creates new neural circuitry that creates, automatic, addictive behaviors - circuitry that may last for a lifetime. *(27)*

What Do We Find Acceptable to Feed Our Kids?

Parents may think by reading the box that the product is healthy because it contains **added** fibre, minerals, and vitamins (which real food doesn't require), however, it doesn't change the fact that these products are loaded with sugar and chemical additives.

Do You Find Eating from Morning 'Till Night Acceptable?

We've been conditioned to think that eating throughout the day is acceptable. Our cultural assumption is that eating late at night is acceptable; eating in the car or while walking down the sidewalk is acceptable. We can't even arrange for a short business meeting without the obligatory coffee and donuts. As one Mom questioned, *"why do I have to bring a snack to a soccer game? This is ridiculous."*

Our food culture facilitates overeating at every turn, and if we're susceptible, it's almost impossible to resist.

Changing What We Find Acceptable

In the last fifty years our diet has changed beyond all recognition; from portion sizes that are out of proportion to a wide acceptance for food with little to no nutritional value.

We need to look differently at what the food industry is trying to sell us and why. We need to look at their advertising with

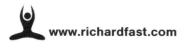

the contempt it deserves. If we stop and analyze any of Big Food's delusional commercials, we can effortlessly take them as a personal insult to our intelligence.

By doing so we'll begin to ask questions such as; why does eating chicken nuggets, and greasy hamburgers make those families in commercials giddy with laughter? Are eating "convenient" frozen dinners ultimately convenient? Are we really so busy, day in and day out, that we cannot find the time to prepare real food?

Our children and we have been conned, addicted and manipulated. The Big Food companies are getting fabulously wealthy by selling us slow-acting poison. Is that acceptable?

Some Closing Thoughts

The title of this book is *OBESITY,* but at heart, it's about health ... all of ours.

Ultimately, each of us is responsible for our own health, and if we don't take personal charge, nothing will change. We

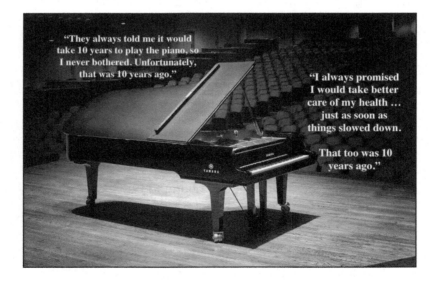

"They always told me it would take 10 years to play the piano, so I never bothered. Unfortunately, that was 10 years ago."

"I always promised I would take better care of my health ... just as soon as things slowed down.

That too was 10 years ago."

simply cannot look outside of ourselves for solutions. However, taking ownership is only effective when we know what actions will work. It begins with awareness.

Having read this book, you know the food you eat is the foundation upon which your health is built. You cannot eat a diet high in ultra-processed foods and be healthy any more than you can chain smoke cigarettes and be healthy. Your diet is key to a life of health and longevity. If you're battling obesity, or being overweight (*remember: overweight and obesity are NOT the same thing*) eliminating ultra-processed food from your diet may not completely solve your weight and obesity challenges, but you *will* lose weight and become healthier in every category of measurable health.

If you dramatically cut back on your consumption of ultra-processed food, you will enjoy noticeable improvements almost immediately.

When we look down our noses at ultra-processed food and equate it with greed, deception, obesity and disease, it becomes much easier to snub this garbage. Let's recognize it for what it is; a carnival of trickery and deceit that generates billions of dollars in profit for Big Food at the expense of our declining health.

And speaking of expense, many people will say they would love to eat real food, but it's too expensive, or they just don't have the time to prepare it.

That may be true for some people, but I'm not sure its valid for most of us. As Michael Pollan points out,

> *... in the last decade or two, we've somehow found the time in the day to spend several hours on the Internet and the money in the budget not only to pay for broadband service but to cover a second phone bill and a new monthly bill for television, formerly free. For the majority of Americans, spending more on better food is less a matter of ability than a priority.*

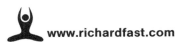

What is the cost of real food?

People get mixed up about food and value. We've been led to equate "more" for "less" as better. We'll choose a super-sized meal of ultra-processed food over a smaller-sized meal of real food. A giant soft drink is thought to be a better value than a similarly priced small glass of fresh juice.

It's true we're getting more, but more of what?

If we look at things from a broader dimension in time, what is the actual cost of those choices? The answer depends on how much value we place on our health.

Perhaps we need to remind ourselves that ultra-processed food is neither *convenient-food* nor is it *food*. If we factor in the cost of our health, it's actually too expensive for anyone.

From a global perspective the cost of our obesity epidemic is immeasurable; the balloon payment for a steady diet of ultra-processed food is still being tabulated, and we're all going to be paying for it.

The prudent perspective is to view your life in terms of health-span rather than lifespan. Each of us needs to make a small investment each day into the most valuable thing we own. Our health is often undervalued ... until we've lost it.

Lifespan is living longer, but there's no glory in being the oldest resident in a long-term care facility. Health-span, on the other hand, is simply choosing to live a lifetime of health.

Fortunately, many of us have that choice.

References

1.Sifferlin, A., "The Weight Loss Trap: Why Your Diet Isn't Working," TIME, Health, June 5, 2017

2. Orpana, H., Berthelot, J., Kaplan, M., Feeny, D., McFarland, B., Ross, N., "BMI and Mortality: Results from a National Longitudinal Study of Canadian Adults," Obesity, January 2010; 18:214–218

3. Yudkin J., "Diet and Coronary Thrombosis. Hypothesis and Fact," Lancet, July 27, 1957; II:155–162

4. Smith, E., "Report on the Sanitary Condition of Tailors in London" In Report of the Medical Officer. London: The Privy Council 1864:416–430 as reported in Domhnall MacAuley, A History of Physical Activity, Health and Medicine, Journal of the Royal Society of Medicine, 1994: 87:32–35

5. Morris, J.N., Crawford, M.D., "Coronary Heart Disease and Physical Activity of Work," British Medical Journal, London: December 20,1958:1486–1495

6. Paffenbarger, R.S. Jr., Blair S.N., Lee, I-M., "A History of Physical Activity, Cardiovascular Health, and Longevity: The Scientific Contribution of Jeremy N. Morris," International Epidemiological Association, 2001; 30:1184–1192

7. Dupen, F., Bauman, A.E., Lin, R,. "The Source of Risk Factor Information for General Practitioners: Is Physical Activity Under-Recognized?" Medical Journal of Australia," Dec 6–20, 1999; 171(11-12): 601–603

8. Thomas L.E., Brynes, A.E., McCarthy, J., Goldstone, A.P., Hajnal, J.V., Saeed, N., Frost, G., Bell, J.D., "Preferential Loss of Visceral Fat Following Aerobic Exercise, Measured by Magnetic Resonance Imaging," Chemistry and Materials Science, LIPIDS, 2000, 35 (7):769–776

9. Revill, J., "Are You a TOFI? (That's Thin on the Outside, Fat Inside), The Observer, Guardian. Dec.10, 2006

10. Ellulu, M. et al., "Obesity and Inflamamation: The Linking Mechanism and the Complications," Arch Med. Sci., 2017 Jun; 13(4):851-863

11. Mullis, R., Blair, S., Arrone, L., Bier, D., Denke, M., Dietz, W., Donato, K., Drewnowski, A., French, S., Howard, B., Robinson, T., Swinburn, B., Weschsler, H., "Prevention Conference VII. "Obesity, a Worldwide Epidemic Related to Heart Disease and Stroke. Group IV: Prevention/Treatment. Circulation, 2004; 110: 484–488

12. Caterson, I., Hubbard, V., Bray, G., Grunstein, R., Hansen, B., Hong, Y., Labarthe, D., Seidell, J.C., Smith, S., "Prevention Conference VII. Obesity, a Worldwide Epidemic Related to Heart Disease and Stroke Group III: Worldwide Comorbidities of Obesity, Circulation, 2004; 110: 476–483

13. Couillard, C., Bergeron, N., Pasco,t A., Almeras, N., Bergeron, J., Tremblay, A., Prud'homme, D., Despres, J.P., "Evidence for Impaired Lipolysis in Abdominally Obese Men: Postprandial Study of Apolipoprotein B-48-and B-100-Containing Lipoproteins," American Journal of Clinical Nutrition, 2002; 76: 311–318

14. Despres, J.P., Coillard, C., Gagnon, J., Bergeron, J., Leon, A., Rao, D., Skinner, J., Wilmore, J., Bouchard, C., "Race, Visceral Adipose Tissue, Plasma Lipids, and Lipoprotein Lipase Activity in Men and Women," (HER-ITAGE). Arteriosclerosis, Thrombosis, and Vascular Biology, 2000; 20:1932–1938

15. Janssen, I., Fortier, A., Hudson, R., Ross, R., "Effects of Energy Restrictive Diet with or Without Exercise on Abdominal Fat, Intermuscular Fat, and Metabolic Risk Factors in Obese Women," Diabetes Care, 2002; 25:431–438

16. Thomas, E.L., Frost, G., Taylor-Robinson, S. D., Bell, J.D., "Excess Body Fat in Obese and Normal-Weight Subjects," Nutrition Research Reviews, 25(1):150-161

17. Kershaw, E.E., Flier, J.S., "Adipose Tissue as An Endocrine Organ," Journal of Clinical Endocrinology and Metabolism, 89(6):2548-56

18. Diehl, M., "The TOFI Phenomenon: Thin Outside, Fat Inside," Democrat & Chronicle, Sept. 10, 2016

19. Frayn, K. N., "Visceral Fat and Insulin Resistance – Causitive or Correlative?" British Journal of Nutrition, (2000), 83 Suppl.1: S71-S77

20. Thomas, E. L., et al, "The Missing Risk: MRI and MRS Phenotyping of Abdominal Adiposity and Ectopic Fat". Obesity. 20(1): 76–87

21. Blair, S.N., Kohl, H.W., Paffenbarger, R.S., Clark, D.G., Cooper, K.H., Gibbons, L.W., "Physical Fitness and All-Cause Mortality, A Prospective Study of Healthy Men and Women," JAMA, 1989; 262:2395–2401

22. Wei, M., Kampert, J., Barlow, C., Nichaman, M., Gibbons, L., Paffenbarger, R., Blari, S., "Relationship Between Low Cardiorespiratory Fitness and Mortality in Normal-Weight, Overweight, and Obese Men," American Medical Association, JAMA, October 27, 1999; Vol 282, No. 16:1547–1553

23. Booth, F.W., Roberts, C.K., Laye, M.J., "Lack of Exercise is a Major Cause of Chronic Diseases," Compr. Physiol., 2012; 2:1143

24. Fiuza-Luces, C., Garatachea, N., Berger, N.A., Lucia, A., "Exercise is the Real Polypill," Physiology (Bethesda). 2013; 28:330

25. Gaesser, G.A., Angadi, S.S., Sawyer, B.J., "Exercise and Diet, Independent of Weight Loss, Improve Cardiometabolic Risk Profile in Overweight and Obese Individuals," Phys. Sportsmed. 2011; 39:87

26. Gaesser, G.A., Tucker, W.J., Jarrett, C., Angadi, S.S., "Fitness versus Fatness: Which Influences Health and Mortality Risk the Most?," American College of Sports Medicine, July 2015, Vol:14:4

27. Kessler, D., "The End of Overeating: Taking Control of the Insatiable American Appetite," Rodale Inc. New York, NY, 2009

28. Staff, "Good Food Gone Bad," Live Science, November, 20, 2006

About Me

My name is Richard Fast. Until I reached my early 50s, I used to be one of "those" people ... the ones who can eat anything they want and never put on a pound. The funny thing is I had never really appreciated my high-revving metabolism – until it began to slow – imperceptibly. I was about 55 when I first suspected that something had changed.

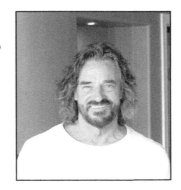

My wife and I love entertaining, especially in the summer when we throw pool parties. One day I was looking at some pictures of a recent party, and I was puzzled to see some chubby guy wearing my bathing suit. When I zoomed in for a closer look, the sickening realization began to sink in, that mystery man was me! How did that happen? When did it happen? How could I – someone who never gained a pound suddenly bear a striking resemblance to a Mcintosh, and I don't mean the computer?

Right then and there, I vowed to lose those extra pounds. So, for the next several months, I tried exercising the weight off, then dieting the weight off, but despite my best intentions, I never quite managed. The scale consistently read 30 pounds "overweight", and for the first time in my life, I began to understand the challenges of weight loss.

So, like the ardent researcher I am, I began investigating weight loss and obesity. Much to my surprise, the more I read, the more I began to understand why dieting and exercise cannot and will not work for most people – because eating too much food wasn't the cause of my obesity, nor is it the cause of most people's obesity. I discovered that obesity is caused by the absurd paradox of being overfed and undernourished. As a society, we have eradicated the problem of hunger (for the most part) in exchange for malnutrition.

I also realized that "food" restriction does not – and cannot – work for healthy weight loss. I eventually learned that our eons-old hunter-gatherer survival mechanisms do not want us to carry any excess fat. So as long as I ate real food – eradicating malnutrition at the cellular level – I began to shed the excess fat, and I never once felt hungry.

I've maintained my desired weight for over ten years. I'm not sharing my story because I intend to tell you to follow the secret of my weight-loss journey; after all, why should you be even remotely interested in my story, or anyone else's for that matter? But I want you to know that I wrote this book because it reveals the foundation of a lifetime of health and vitality. And what's more, there is nothing you need to buy, nor is there any diet you need to follow. This book will help you find what works for you and it's all based on maximizing your health – first and foremost.

As an entrepreneur, I'm the creator of MindTrap® games and more than 20 other puzzles and toys that have sold millions of copies worldwide. I am also an American Council of Exercise certified trainer, Weight Management Specialist and Health & Wellness coach.

Through intense research, practical knowledge, and first-hand application - I have discovered how to tap more energy and vitality in my 60s than at any other time in my life. It's my passion to help you achieve your best health as well.

My wife Michele and I live in Ontario, Canada and share a mutual passion for health, fitness, and food.

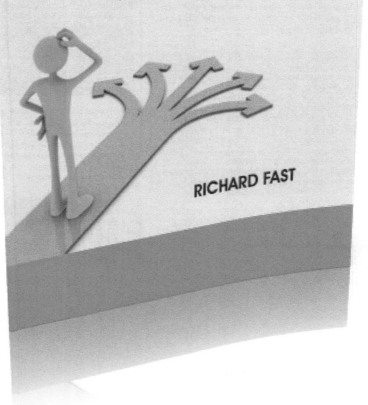

The Challenge
of Choice

... how to make a "good" decision
when it *REALLY* matters!

RICHARD FAST

Have you ever made an important decision with total confidence, only to see it become a complete disaster? Or perhaps you've made a critical decision in haste, hoping things would work out?

Why do we frequently make crucial decisions based on false confidence and wishful thinking?

... because the human brain makes many time–saving assumptions to navigate our modern world, resulting in faulty insights and delusional beliefs without the slightest awareness from our conscious self.

Surprisingly (or not), *everyone* is susceptible to making bad decisions, regardless of our intelligence, I.Q., or level of education, because we *all* mistake "feeling right" with "being right" resulting in decisions that are irrationally void of logic and reason.

This book will challenge the way you think about making critical decisions by taking you on a fascinating journey into the inner workings of the human mind.

Through quizzes, exercises, and many real-world examples, you will discover how your decisions are really made and why you can be most vulnerable to decisional error, precisely when your confidence is at its highest. You'll see how you can easily detect and overcome the common cognitive illusions that inevitably lead to poor choices and bad judgment.

When it comes to making critical decisions, most people assume they won't know if they've made a "good" decision until they see the outcome, but this line of thinking is entirely backward.

If you cannot make a critical decision with 100% confidence before you know the outcome, then it's NOT decision-making – it's hoping, gambling and wishful thinking!

When you understand how your mind really works (it's not how you think) you will develop the discipline to follow this book's simple decision-making formula – and that means making those critical, potentially life-changing decisions with confidence and certainty.

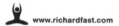 www.richardfast.com

ISBN 978-0-9879193-6-6

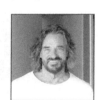

Made in the USA
Coppell, TX
25 August 2023

20754266R00070